Lymphoedema

Lymphoedema Care

Mary Woods

Clinical Nurse Specialist/Head of
Lymphoedema Services, MSc. BSc.
(Hons) RGN Onc. Cert.

Blackwell
Publishing

Blackwell Publishing editorial offices:
Blackwell Publishing Ltd, 9600 Garsington Road, Oxford OX4 2DQ, UK
Tel: +44 (0)1865 776868
Blackwell Publishing Inc., 350 Main Street, Malden, MA 02148-5020, USA
Tel: +1 781 388 8250
Blackwell Publishing Asia Pty Ltd, 550 Swanston Street, Carlton, Victoria 3053, Australia
Tel: +61 (0)3 8359 1011

First published 2007 by Blackwell Publishing Ltd

ISBN: 978-1-4051-4628-9

Library of Congress Cataloging-in-Publication Data
Woods, Mary, 1957–
Lymphoedema care / Mary Woods.
p. ; cm.
Includes bibliographical references and index.
ISBN-13: 978-1-4051-4628-9 (pbk. : alk. paper)
1. Lymphedema. 2. Lymphedema—Treatment. I. Title.
[DNLM: 1. Lymphedema. 2. Lymphedema—therapy. WH 700 W896 2007]
RC646.3.W66 2007
616.4′2—dc22
2007020582

A catalogue record for this title is available from the British Library

Set in 10/12.5pt Palatino
by Graphicraft Limited, Hong Kong
Printed and bound in Singapore
by Fabulous Printers Pte Ltd

For further information on Blackwell Publishing, visit our website:
www.blackwellnursing.com

Contents

Foreword

Lymphoedema is perceived as an unimportant condition, for which there is no satisfactory or available treatment. This state of affairs understandably upsets suffers. Nevertheless lymphoedema care has progressed considerably in the last 25 years, although much remains to be done, particularly in the education of health care professionals, as to what can be done to benefit patients.

The introduction of Decongestive Lymphoedema Treatment (DLT) and its specific components including compression, exercise, massage and skin care in the early 1980s brought a rational and constructive approach to lymphoedema care. Previously treatment was rather cursory. Patients were provided with compression hosiery, more in hope than expectation, and told that lymphoedema was a small price to pay for the cure of their cancer.

In the UK in 1987 the first dedicated and comprehensive lymphoedema clinic for cancer patients was established at the Royal Marsden Hospital, London utilising the technique of DLT. Mary Woods joined the lymphoedema team soon after and has been head of lymphoedema services for more than 10 years. As a result she has gained enormous experience in the care of cancer patients with lymphoedema and has trained countless numbers of therapists. Therefore she is well placed to inform on lymphoedema care, particularly in the cancer setting. This book brings together that wealth of experience and is directed at healthcare professionals who encounter cancer related lymphoedema. It is written and presented in an effective and practical manner with an appreciation of the psychological impact of lymphoedema, an aspect in which Mary has had a particular interest. The information provided is equally essential reading for professionals working in primary care as it is for those working in oncology.

Peter Mortimer
August 2007

Preface

The development of lymphoedema in a limb heralds the onset of a chronic condition which can require significant personal and professional resources in order to keep the swelling under control during what may be a lifetime of awareness. The intention of this book is to equip health-care professionals with the necessary knowledge and skills to identify those at risk of the development of lymphoedema and enable them to provide advice and information to patients concerning the management of mild, uncomplicated lymphoedema in order to minimise the risk of problematic swelling developing.

As cancer becomes more prevalent and patients live longer with their disease, health-care professionals working within a wide range of health-care settings will encounter patients with, or at risk of the development of, lymphoedema. Although the focus of this book is predominantly on secondary, cancer-related lymphoedema, the contents will also be invaluable to health-care professionals caring for patients with primary lymphoedema who continually struggle to find help and information for their condition. This book will help to address the gaps in knowledge that still exist about the care required by this group of patients.

The book consists of 12 chapters, leading the reader from an outline of what lymphoedema is to a consideration of who is at risk of its development and how to identify lymphoedema. Aspects of assessment and important areas of care for all patients, whether swelling in the limb is present or not, are then discussed and the book concludes by considering what it is like to live with lymphoedema and providing an outline of complications requiring more specialist intervention.

A comprehensive but focused approach has been used with the intention of providing core knowledge and skills regarding the management of lymphoedema for a wide group of professionals. It is hoped that this approach highlights the importance of this area of care and how, rather than being just for specialists, it can be the responsibility of all health-care professionals.

Mary Woods
April 2007

Acknowledgements

I am indebted to the many patients with lymphoedema from whom I have been privileged to learn so much and without whom this book would not have arisen. Thanks are due to Beth and Katharine at Blackwell Publishing for their guidance along the journey and to my colleagues for their encouragement. I also wish to thank those who have provided permission for me to include photographs within this book. Finally, special thanks are due to Robin, Alex and Bryony who provided endless patience, support and understanding whilst enduring many hours of my absence from family life during the completion of this challenge.

The case studies at the end of each chapter have been included to highlight aspects of lymphoedema management and are based upon patients whose care I have been involved with. Their names and some of the details have been changed to protect the identity of those concerned.

Dedicated to my mother Nora

1 What is Lymphoedema?

Introduction

Lymphoedema affects millions of people worldwide, but has different causes for its development. The most common cause of lymphoedema in modern western society is cancer and its treatment, whilst in tropical and subtropical climates, transmission of the filarial worm through the vector of mosquito bites leads to lymphatic filariasis. A congenital abnormality of the lymphatic system due to underdevelopment of the lymphatic system is called primary lymphoedema, the onset of which may be gradual or sudden and is often delayed until teenage years or later life.

In order to understand the management of a patient with lymphoedema, an understanding of the cause of the swelling is essential. The aim of this chapter is to explain the principles of oedema formation and why lymphoedema, as one type of oedema, may develop.

Learning objectives

At the end of this chapter the reader will be able to:

- outline the structure and function of the normal lymphatic system
- describe the physiological causes of oedema
- describe the term lymphoedema and the different types that are identified
- describe the reasons for the development of lymphoedema
- outline how lymphoedema is diagnosed.

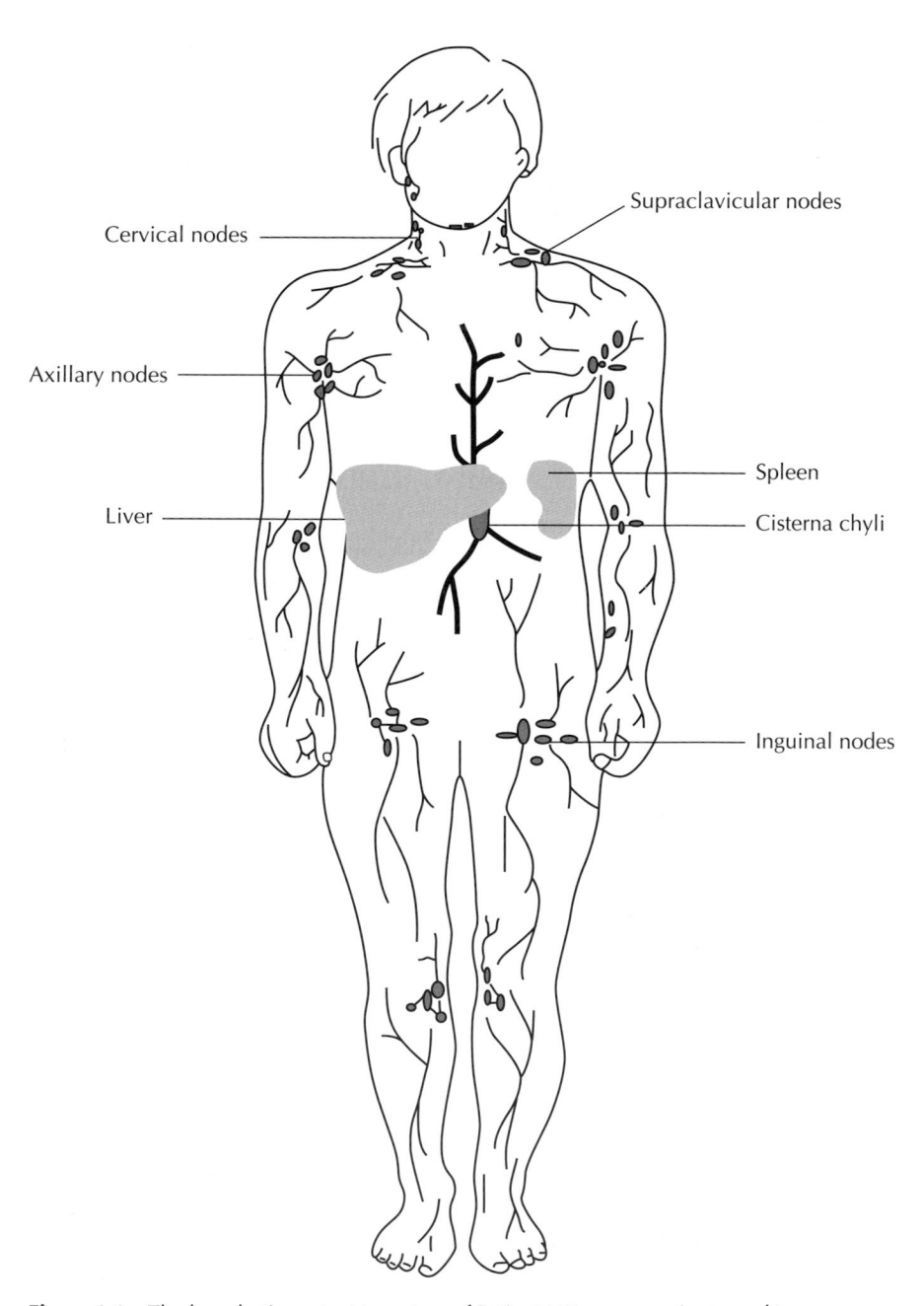

Figure 1.1 The lymphatic system (courtesy of Patient UK, www.patient.co.uk).

The lymphatic system

The lymphatic system is a one-way drainage system leading fluid from the tissues of the body to the veins in the neck. Lymphatic vessels are present in all tissues except the brain and bone marrow. Tiny lymph vessels converge to form larger vessels which pass through a series of lymph nodes to drain into two ducts, the thoracic duct and the right lymphatic duct, and finally empty into the venous system. A diagram of the lymphatic system can be seen in Figure 1.1.

Structure

- *Initial lymphatics.* These are blind-ended tubes which are found in the connective tissue spaces and are bathed by intracellular tissue fluid. The initial lymphatics are composed of a single layer of thin, flat endothelial cells with flaps which close when the vessel is full and lymph then moves into the adjacent lymph vessel. The movement of fluid in the initial lymphatics is dependent upon changes in local tissue pressure and muscle activity in the body rather than valves which are not found in the initial lymphatics.
- *Larger lymph vessels.* These delicate vessels are surrounded by smooth muscle cells and contain valves formed of thin layers of fibrous tissue covered by endothelium which ensure a unidirectional flow of lymph away from the tissues. The valves are most numerous close to the lymph nodes and in the upper extremity of the body. The larger lymph vessels have their own blood and nerve supply and contract actively to propel lymph. Movement of lymph in these larger vessels is influenced by skeletal muscle contraction, peristalsis in the gut and intrathoracic pressure changes in the lungs during breathing.
- *Lymph nodes.* The lymph nodes are surrounded by a fibrous capsule and have an internal honeycomb structure. They have a small, bean or kidney-shaped appearance and are situated in groups of various sizes within the lymphatic vessels. Lymphocytes within the nodes act like filters, collecting and destroying bacteria and viruses. Lymph nodes range in size from a few mm to 1–2 cm in their normal state, but may become enlarged due to tumour or infection. The number of lymph nodes in the body ranges from 500 to 1500 with the largest clusters found in the head and neck region, axillae, groin, pelvis and abdomen. Figure 1.2 shows the structure of a lymph node.
- *Lymph.* Lymph is found in closed lymphatic vessels as a transparent, colourless fluid with a similar composition to blood plasma. It contains plasma proteins, dead cells, organic matter, foreign bodies and fat from

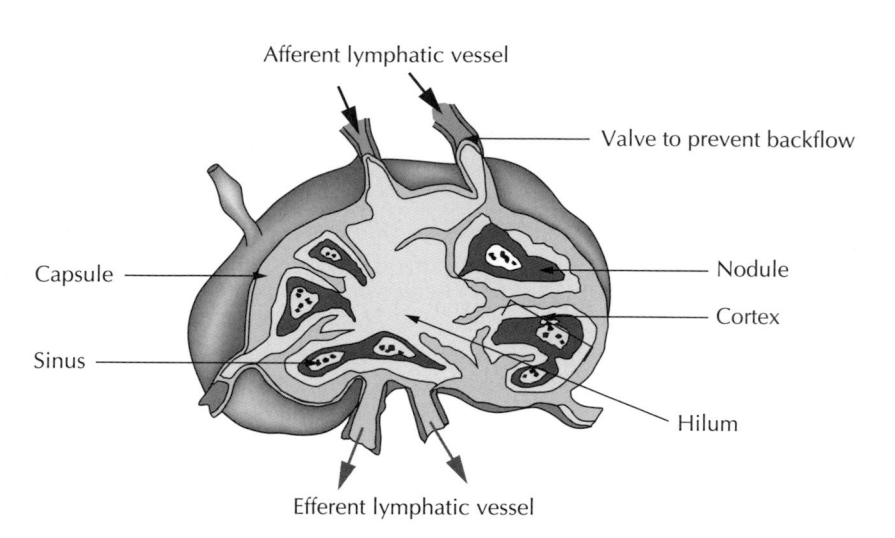

Afferent lymphatic vessel

Valve to prevent backflow

Capsule

Nodule

Cortex

Sinus

Hilum

Efferent lymphatic vessel

Figure 1.2   The structure of a lymph node.
Source: Wikipedia.

the intestine. Lymph circulates to the lymph node via afferent lymphatic vessels, draining into the node just beneath the capsule in a space called the subcapsular sinus. Foreign bodies are trapped here and the lymph is filtered before leaving the lymph node via the efferent lymphatic vessel.

Functions of the lymphatics

The lymphatics have three important functions in the body.

- A waste disposal function, reabsorbing plasma proteins and absorbing cell debris and particulate matter.
- An immunological function, absorbing microorganisms and defending against infections.
- The maintenance of tissue fluid levels, returning excess filtered fluid and protein to the blood.

The physiological causes of oedema

Fluid and protein continuously leak out of capillaries and enter the interstitial compartment of the tissues to form interstitial fluid. The fluid then enters the smallest lymphatic vessels and is transported away by the lymphatic system. After filtering and the removal of some water at the lymph nodes, the fluid re-enters the blood via a connection between the lymphatics and the large veins at the base of the neck.

An equilibrium is normally maintained between tissue fluid formation and reabsorption in the body which is dependent upon hydrostatic and osmotic pressures, known as Starling's forces, across the capillary wall.

- Hydrostatic pressure is the pressure in the blood capillaries which causes fluid to be filtered outwards from the blood to the interstitial spaces.
- Osmotic pressure occurs in the blood due to the plasma proteins which suck fluid back into the capillaries.

The membrane of the vascular capillary is semi-permeable, allowing the blood pressure in the arterial end of the capillary to drive fluid (water and some proteins) outwards from the blood to the interstitial spaces, causing the formation of interstitial fluid. Interstitial fluid contains very little protein and the high concentration of plasma protein in the blood produces osmotic pressure, which sucks the water back into the capillary at the venous end of the capillary. The blood pressure is higher at the arterial end of the capillary than the osmotic pressure in the interstitium and so fluid is forced out into the tissue. However, at the venous end of the capillary, the blood pressure has dropped below the osmotic pressure and so fluid is drawn back into the capillary (Green 1978).

Any change can affect fluid levels in the tissues and when the volume of fluid entering the interstitial compartment of the tissues is greater than the rate at which it is drained, oedema appears. Oedema can be temporary and resolve once the causative factor is corrected.

The physiological factors associated with the development of oedema can be classified into four groups.

Increased permeability of the capillary walls

This is due to a release of histamine and other substances which result from burns, trauma and allergic reactions leading to inflammation and infection.

Decreased plasma osmotic pressure

This problem is found in malnutrition, liver disease, profuse serous drainage and haemorrhage. A low albumin level in the blood may result from decreased albumin synthesis or nutritional protein deficiency and result in lower limb and ankle swelling.

Increased plasma hydrostatic pressure

This causes fluid to be squeezed into the tissues, due to circulatory over-load. This type of oedema is commonly seen in conditions such as heart failure (due to salt and water retention), kidney failure (due to salt and water retention) and excessive infusions of isotonic or other sodium-containing solutions. It may also result from venous obstruction, venous disease or immobility where continuous dependency of the legs leads to increased capillary pressure related to increased venous pressure.

Reduced lymphatic system transport capacity

A reduction in the lymphatic system transport capacity can develop when damage or obstruction occurs in the lymphatic system. This reduces the available drainage routes for lymph fluid and lymphoedema can appear. It can occur following cancer-related treatment in lymph node areas of the body or when advanced or recurrent tumour obstructs lymph node regions. Lymphoedema is a chronic, permanent swelling of the whole or part of a limb due to damage sustained to the lymphatic system and the accumulation of interstitial fluid in the tissues.

Types of lymphoedema and their development

Lymphoedema is classified as primary or secondary, terms which refer to the cause of its development.

Primary lymphoedema

Primary lymphoedema arises from an abnormality occurring within the lymphatic system. Browse (2003) indicates that alternative titles for the term 'primary lymphoedema' have included:

- idiopathic, indicating that the lymphoedema is of unknown origin
- intrinsic, indicating that the lymphoedema is due to an abnormality within the lymphatic system
- spontaneous, indicating that the lymphoedema occurred without intervention.

Kinmouth (1982) classified this type of oedema according to the age of onset of the swelling, as highlighted in Table 1.1, and in terms of the lympho-graphic appearance of lymph vessels established during lymphography scanning procedures, which are highlighted in Table 1.2.

Table 1.1 Classification of primary lymphoedema according to age (adapted from Kinmouth 1982).

Classification of primary lymphoedema	Age at onset of lymphoedema
Congenital	Present at birth or within two years
Praecox	Appearing after birth but before 35 years of age
Tarda	Appearing after the age of 35 years

Table 1.2 Classification of primary lymphoedema according to lymphographic appearances (adapted from Kinmouth 1982).

Classification of primary lymphoedema	Lymphographic appearance of lymphatic vessels
Aplasia	No collecting lymph vessels detected
Hypoplasia	A lower than normal number of lymph vessels detected
Hyperplasia	An increased number of lymphatic vessels detected

Primary lymphoedema is also associated with some chromosomal and single gene abnormalities which result in a wide range of lymphatic abnormalities and differing presentations. These are classified as genetically determined abnormalities or acquired abnormalities and include clinical syndromes such as Turner's syndrome, Noonan's syndrome, Klippel–Trenaunay syndrome and Milroy's disease.

A more recent classification system for primary lymphoedema included these known abnormalities of the lymphatic system and described the development of the condition according to genetically determined abnormalities or acquired abnormalities (Browse 2003). The classification of primary lymphoedema continues to be debated. As more is understood about different clinical manifestations and more complex techniques for the investigation of lymphatic vessels are developed, further classifications will emerge. A greater understanding of the cause of primary lymphoedema will, in the future, facilitate more effective treatment.

Secondary lymphoedema

Secondary lymphoedema arises from the influence of an external factor which affects the function of the lymphatic system. Keeley (2000) identified four categories pertaining to the cause of secondary lymphoedema.

- Infection
- Inflammation
- Trauma
- Cancer and its treatment

Infection

Filariasis

The most common cause of secondary lymphoedema worldwide is infection due to lymphatic filariasis. A parasitic, tissue-dwelling, thread-like worm enters the body through the vector of a mosquito, to live and develop in the lymph glands and vessels. The adult male lives for approximately six years and during its life cycle the female worm releases millions of immature worms which circulate in the blood. The developing worms, which can grow to between 40 and 100 mm in length, coupled with the associated inflammatory reaction to their presence, gradually impede the flow of lymph through the lymphatic vessels they occupy, to cause lymphoedema.

Although confined to the geographical areas of India, Africa, South Asia and parts of Central and South America, lymphatic filariasis affects millions of people and is considered by the World Health Organisation to be the fourth most common cause of permanent disability worldwide (WHO 1998). The disease is prevalent among poor communities where inadequate sanitation, stagnant water and family crowding among dwellings encourage mosquitoes to breed in dirty water and transmit the disease from person to person.

The infection is usually acquired in childhood but the symptoms can take years to appear as the worms grow in size. Successful elimination of the filariatic worm is dependent upon the administration of effective medication to whole populations rather than individuals alone and recognising lymphatic filariasis as a disease of poverty, public health programmes have targeted populations with free antifilarial drugs. Those already infected cannot be cured but the administration of two oral drugs once a year for at least five years will kill the immature worms in an infected person's blood and prevent transmission of the disease by the mosquito from person to person.

Lymphatic filariasis carries a heavy social burden. It exacerbates poverty as those affected become physically unable to lead a normal working life (Wegesa et al. 1979) and the visible swelling leads to social stigma. Figure 1.3 illustrates chronic lymphatic filariasis. Damage to the lymphatic system can cause fluid to collect in the genitals, leading to a poor self-image and social isolation. Males affected in this way suffer physical

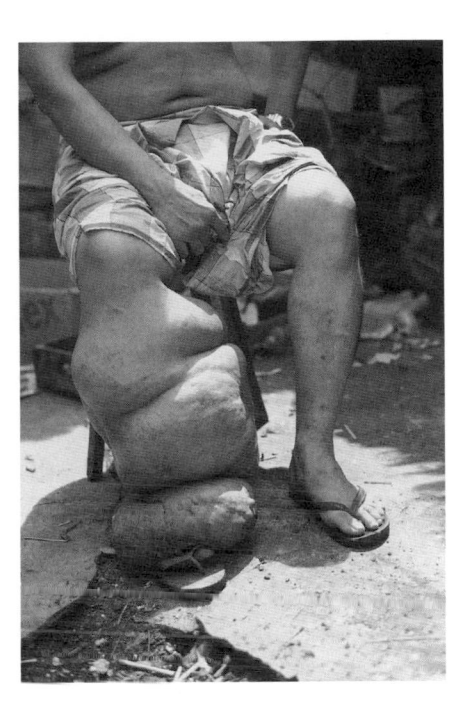

Figure 1.3   Chronic lymphatic filariasis (courtesy of Dr Ted Bianco/The Wellcome Trust).

limitations and women with lymphoedema due to filariasis are often considered undesirable and find it impossible to gain the security of marriage (WHO 1998).

Bacterial infection
Repeated bacterial infection involving the superficial layers of the skin and the subcutaneous tissues can cause local signs of inflammation and subsequent damage to the lymphatic channels through fibrosis. Keeley (2000) suggests that patients who develop lymphoedema following bacterial infections may already have a previously unrecognised lymphatic abnormality, placing them at risk of its development.

Inflammation

Lymphoedema may develop as a complication of several inflammatory processes which arise without the presence of infection. Chronic conditions such as arthritis, psoriasis and dermatitis cause inflammatory changes to occur within the skin lymphatics. These then become obstructed with debris from the inflammatory process, placing the individual at risk of the development of lymphoedema. Treatment for the condition is aimed at reducing the inflammation.

Trauma

Function of the lymphatic vessels and glands may be impeded by trauma caused by accidental or self-inflicted injury and some surgical procedures. Trauma may occur as a result of burns or severe wounds with extensive tissue loss. Lymphoedema has been observed in some psychiatric illnesses where self-harm occurs most frequently following the prolonged application of a tourniquet around a limb (Mortimer 2003).

Cancer and its treatment

The most common cause of lymphoedema in modern western society is cancer and its treatment. The surgical excision of regional lymphatic nodes is regarded as an essential procedure to provide prognostic information for many types of cancer, but damage to the lymphatic vessels or a reduction in their number as a result of the surgery can lead to the development of lymphoedema. Radiation therapy, used to destroy cancer cells, can also damage normal lymph cells within the irradiated area and inflict damage to the lymph channels. A combination of surgery and radiation treatment to lymph node areas can cause significant damage to the lymph channels.

The presence of malignant cells due to secondary deposits in the lymph vessels must also be considered in a patient with a cancer diagnosis who has developed lymphoedema.

Diagnosing lymphoedema

A diagnosis of lymphoedema can be made without the patient undergoing medical investigations and is usually made following a detailed medical history and clinical examination. Where a diagnosis is unclear, images of the lymphatic vessels can be obtained following the injection of a radioactive medium into the subcutaneous tissues. The transport of the medium via the lymphatic vessels in this procedure, known as lymphoscintigraphy, can be followed by an external gamma camera to provide information about lymphatic function.

The following case scenarios illustrate differing causes for the development of oedema.

Case Scenario 1

John is a 68-year-old retired factory worker with a history of bronchitis. He gets breathless when he walks too quickly to the local shops and this makes him feel dizzy. His doctor keeps an eye on his blood pressure when he attends the surgery every few months, because it has a tendency to be a little higher than normal.

John and his wife manage at home but need help in their big garden. One day part of a tree falls following a heavy wind and John has to work hard to move it from the shed roof where it has landed. He gets very breathless and has to rest regularly. That evening he is very tired and he notices that his ankles are swollen. He spends the evening watching television and is too tired the next day to do much except potter around the house. A few days later, his wife becomes concerned because John is still very breathless and his swollen ankles are bigger. She calls the doctor to arrange an appointment.

Consider John's history and reflect on what you think may be the cause of his swollen ankles.

- What physiological processes may cause ankle swelling to develop?
- Consider any background reading you may have completed and reflect upon how you could explain to John why he has swollen ankles.

The history suggests that John has swollen ankles because of congestive cardiac failure in which the heart is not pumping well enough to meet the body's demand for oxygen and congestion occurs in the lungs. Swollen ankles can be one of the first signs of this developing.

An increase of pressure in the blood vessels to the lungs causes pressure to back up in the right side of the heart. Increased plasma hydrostatic pressure leads to swelling in the feet and ankles.

John and his wife need to know that John's heart is not pumping efficiently any more and pressure building up in the heart causes John to become breathless and his ankles to become swollen. John needs to work within his limits and not overexert himself. He also needs to have his blood pressure recorded regularly so that his medication can be adjusted appropriately.

Case Scenario 2

Hazel is a 64-year-old widowed lady who lives alone in a retirement flat. Hazel is rather overweight and does not go out very much because she finds it difficult to walk far. Over recent months she has been unwell with a chest infection and has needed more help at home than normal. She spends most of the day sitting in the chair looking out into the garden and since she developed the chest infection, she has found it easier to stay in the chair at night because she can breathe more easily. Her nephew notices that she has developed swelling in her legs and one day the skin looks so shiny and fragile that he thinks the legs may burst.

Consider Hazel's history and reflect on what you think may be the cause of her swollen legs.

- What physiological processes may cause the swelling to develop?
- Consider any background reading you may have completed and reflect upon how you could explain to Hazel and her nephew why she has swollen legs.

Hazel may have developed swollen legs for two reasons. As she has been unwell, it is possible that she has not been eating as well as normal and therefore may have developed a low albumin level in the blood. This can result in swelling of both feet and legs in which the skin becomes stretched and fragile. It is more likely, however, that Hazel has developed swollen legs due to immobility and prolonged dependency of the legs through sitting during the day in her chair and also sleeping in the chair at night. The capillary filtration rate becomes raised due to increased venous pressure as the muscle pump remains inactive. Swelling appears in both feet and legs with the skin appearing to be very thin and fragile.

Hazel should be encouraged to elevate her legs at heart level while she is sitting in her chair and to try to sleep in her bed at night with pillows to support her. She should also be encouraged to try taking short walks regularly to encourage the muscle pump in the legs to become active which will assist in reducing venous pressure.

Conclusion

There are many reasons for the development of oedema and an understanding of the physiological processes involved is essential in order to identify a causative factor. Although this book will focus on lymphoedema, this chapter has highlighted some of the many other reasons why oedema can occur in order to eliminate their influence when caring for the patient with lymphoedema.

References

Browse N. (2003) Aetiology and classifications of lymphoedema. In: N. Browse, K. Burnard and P. Mortimer (eds) *Diseases of the Lymphatics*. Arnold/Oxford University Press, New York, pp. 151–6.

Green J.H. (1978) *Basic Clinical Physiology*, 3rd edn. Oxford University Press, Oxford.

Keeley V. (2000) Classification of lymphoedema. In: R. Twycross, K. Jenns and J. Todd (eds) *Lymphoedema*. Radcliffe Medical Press, Oxford, pp. 22–43.

Kinmouth J. (1982) *The Lymphatics*, 2nd edn. Arnold, London.

Mortimer P. (2003) Medical and physical treatment. In: N. Browse, K. Burnard and P. Mortimer (eds) *Diseases of the Lymphatics*. Arnold/Oxford University Press, New York, pp. 165–8.

Wegesa P., McMahon J.E., Abam D.E., Hamilton P.J.S., Marshall T.F. and Vaughan J.P. (1979) Tanzania filariasis project: survey methodology and clinical manifestations of bancroftian filariasis. *Acta Tropica*, **36**(4): 369–77.

World Health Organisation (1998) *World Health Report*. World Health Organisation, Geneva.

2 Risk Factors for the Development of Secondary Lymphoedema

Introduction

Lymphoedema developing as a result of lymphatic insufficiency or damage following treatment for cancer does not always occur and many people find that their lymph drainage is unaffected by the treatment they have undergone. When lymphoedema does occur, factors involved in the development and appearance of the swelling can often be identified and form the basis for education of the patient and the successful management of early swelling. The *cause* of lymphoedema development differs from identifiable *risks* associated with its appearance and *trigger factors* which may initiate its development. By identifying these factors at an early stage, before swelling develops, and alerting the patient to simple adaptive behaviours aimed at caring for their 'at-risk' limb, the possibility that swelling may develop can be reduced.

Studies have estimated the number of patients who have developed lymphoedema following treatment for cancer (Kissin et al. 1986, Mortimer et al. 1996, Querci della Rovere et al. 2003, Ryan et al. 2003, Williams et al. 2005) and others attempt to estimate those who are at risk (Clark et al. 2005).

This chapter will consider the estimated incidence of lymphoedema and factors thought to be involved in its development.

Learning objectives

At the end of this chapter the reader will be able to:

- demonstrate knowledge of the incidence of lymphoedema
- discuss risk factors for the development of secondary lymphoedema

- identify disease, treatment and patient-related factors that may place a patient at risk of the development of secondary lymphoedema
- demonstrate knowledge of relevant studies relating to risk factors for the development of secondary lymphoedema.

The incidence of lymphoedema

Filariasis

Filariasis is endemic in the tropical regions of Asia, Africa and South America with an estimated 120 million people infected in at least 80 nations of the world (WHO 1998). One-third of those affected live in India, one-third in Africa and the remaining third live in South Asia, the Western Pacific and parts of Central and South America (Ottensen et al. 1997).

Cancer-related secondary lymphoedema

The development of secondary lymphoedema in any part of the body is often observed first by the patient. Once a health-care professional is consulted, advice regarding the management of the lymphoedema should be given, whilst the lymphoedema remains mild and uncomplicated. However, many patients with lymphoedema, particularly non-cancer related lymphoedema, are known to experience difficulty accessing advice because among health-care professionals knowledge of how to manage the swelling is variable and specialist services, where advice and treatment is available, tend to be poorly distributed.

Current treatment and research are primarily focused on those with cancer-related lymphoedema while non-cancer related lymphoedema remains less well recognised by health-care professionals. Sitzia et al. (1998), in a study of 27 lymphoedema clinics in the UK, reported that 80% of patients had cancer-related lymphoedema and that patients with non-cancer related lymphoedema had suffered the condition disproportionately longer than the cancer-related group. Hardy & Taylor (1999) suggested that 25% of the population of lymphoedema patients may have non-cancer related lymphoedema and that these patients were disadvantaged in obtaining access to treatment due to a lack of understanding of their condition and imposed funding limitations in providing the advice required.

The magnitude of the problem of breast cancer-related arm lymphoedema has been estimated by Mortimer et al. (1996) in a prevalence study which suggests that as many as 28% of women may develop lymphoedema at some time following their breast cancer treatment. Querci della

Rovere et al. (2003) considered lymphoedema a common complication of axillary surgery with mild, uncomplicated lymphoedema affecting an estimated 27% of patients. The incidence of lymphoedema occurring in the leg has not been widely reported but Werngren-Elgstrom & Lidman (1994), in a study of 54 women who had received treatment for cancer of the cervix, reported that 41% of the women developed measurable lymphoedema of the leg.

Williams et al. (2005) state that definitions of the presence of lymphoedema vary and that there is a lack of sound incidence and prevalence data. Incidence of the condition, indicating the number of patients developing the condition, provides valuable information on which to plan the provision of care, whilst prevalence indicates the long-term burden of the condition. As incidence and prevalence data are difficult to confirm, efforts to minimise the risk of lymphoedema developing among new patients are supported primarily by physiological arguments.

Risk factors for the development of lymphoedema

Filariasis

The WHO estimates that there are a billion people at risk of developing lymphatic filariasis. The rapid, unplanned growth of cities in countries where communities exist in poverty creates numerous breeding sites for the mosquitoes that transmit the disease (WHO 1998).

Short-term travellers to areas where filariasis is endemic are at low risk for this infection but if travel is for an extended period of time, exposure to infected mosquitoes places the individual at risk of acquiring the infection and appropriate precautions should be taken. Most infections of filariasis in westernised countries occur among immigrants from endemic countries.

Cancer-related secondary lymphoedema

The evidence base for defining which procedures or events are likely to place an individual at risk of developing cancer-related lymphoedema is the subject of much discussion and debate. Although largely based on anecdotal evidence of incidence supported by a physiological background, it is possible to identify a wide range of factors which are considered potential risks for the development of lymphoedema, some of which have been studied in more detail.

These can be considered within three main areas which are discussed here and summarised in Table 2.1.

Table 2.1   Risk factors for the development of lymphoedema.

Disease-related factors		
Cancer status	Cancer stage at diagnosis	
Treatment-related factors		
Surgery:	Radiotherapy:	Postoperative events:
Involving lymph nodes	Involving lymph nodes	● Seroma formation
in the axilla, groin or	in the axilla, breast or groin	● Cording
pelvis		● Thrombosis
		● Venepuncture
		● Infection
Patient-related factors		
Concurrent medical	Demographic issues:	Skin conditions:
conditions and	● Age	● Psoriasis
medications	● Weight	● Eczema
	● Activities involving the limb	● Trauma

- Disease-related factors
- Treatment-related factors
- Patient-related factors

Disease-related factors

At the time of diagnosis, treatment for the patient with cancer may involve excision of the tumour and removal or sampling of the regional lymph nodes in order to establish the status of the disease. Decisions can then be made concerning the medical management necessary. A number of authors have suggested that the presence of positive regional lymph nodes at the time of surgery is predictive of an increased risk of lymphoedema development (Herd-Smith et al. 2001, Kissin et al. 1986, Querci della Rovere et al. 2003, Sener et al. 2001).

Lymphoedema can also develop as a result of metastatic tumour in lymph node areas causing an obstruction in the lymphatic channels and the appearance of swelling. Treatment to reduce the size of the tumour can have a positive impact on the resulting lymphoedema.

Treatment-related factors

Many patients with cancer are at risk of developing lymphoedema as a result of their cancer treatment. Surgery or radiotherapy to any lymph node area can reduce the number of functioning lymphatic vessels in the area and interrupt the transport capacity of remaining lymphatics. As this interruption is permanent, lymphoedema can develop at any time and may be

Table 2.2 Types of cancer in which lymph node intervention occurs.

Breast cancer	Axillary lymph nodes Sentinel lymph node
Sarcoma	Inguinal lymph nodes
Melanoma	Regional lymph nodes may include axillary or inguinal lymph nodes
Head and neck cancers	Supraclavicular lymph nodes or cervical lymph nodes
Pelvic cancers, e.g. bladder, prostate, cervix, uterus	Internal and external iliac lymph nodes and inguinal lymph nodes

triggered by a number of factors that will be discussed. Table 2.2 illustrates the different types of cancer that may require lymph node intervention.

Surgery

The degree of surgery to lymph node areas has been reported to influence the later development of lymphoedema (Querci della Rovere et al. 2003) and over recent years modifications have been made to the diagnostic techniques involved in establishing disease status in order to minimise complications of lymphoedema. Sentinel lymph node biopsy, involving the identification and biopsy of the first node to which the lymph drains from a breast tumour, is a proposed option to axillary dissection (Pressman 1998). Although it still involves lymph node intervention and therefore carries a risk of subsequent lymphoedema development, sentinel lymph node biopsy is thought to have a lower risk of lymphoedema development than axillary node dissection for patients with breast cancer (Golshan et al. 2003).

Radiotherapy

The combination of surgery and radiotherapy to the axilla following a breast cancer diagnosis is widely reported as a risk factor for the development of lymphoedema (Kwan et al. 2002, Mortimer et al. 1996, Segerstrom et al. 1992). However, the degree of risk may be related to the dose of radiotherapy, the reaction of the skin and any fibrosis that subsequently develops in the tissues.

The effects of radiotherapy can be considered as short term or long term. Skin breakdown and inflammation will resolve once the treatment is completed, but tissue fibrosis and destruction of the brachial nerve can become evident many years following treatment and be associated with the development of lymphoedema.

Postoperative events

Following surgery in lymph node areas, a number of postoperative events are considered to be identifiable risk factors for the development of lymphoedema, but research in these areas is limited. As lymphoedema may develop many years following treatment, postoperative events can be unclear or become forgotten.

- *Seroma formation.* The accumulation of fluid in the surgical wound requiring frequent aspiration in the weeks following surgery is considered to indicate impaired lymph drainage. Tadych & Donegan (1987) noted an association between high volumes of postoperative wound drainage and lymphoedema in a retrospective study of patients following mastectomy whilst Compton (1997) was unable to establish a causal link between the development of seromas and lymphoedema of the arm.
- *Cording.* Tender cord-like structures of varying thickness can develop postoperatively and extend from the axilla along the inner aspect of the arm. The cords can cause pain when the arm is extended and are thought to result from thrombosis or inflammation of the local lymphatic channels (Stanton et al. 1996). The relationship of cording to the development of lymphoedema is unclear, but inflammation associated with the presence of cords can result in arm swelling of an acute nature. Exercises to stretch the cords can be successful in achieving a full range of movement within a few months and the swelling frequently resolves as the cords disappear.
- *Thrombosis.* A thrombosis developing in the axillary or deep veins of the leg can initiate an acute inflammatory response and the development of swelling in the limb. The thrombosis can lead to increased venous pressure and a subsequent increase in lymph load but the symptoms usually resolve with anticoagulation treatment. When swelling becomes chronic following a thrombosis, it is termed post-thrombotic syndrome and management is similar to that for lymphoedema.
- *Venepuncture.* Therapeutic access to veins in a limb where there is impaired lymph drainage may cause damage to surrounding tissues and result in increased capillary filtration. Smith (1998) reported a positive association between venous access of an 'at-risk' arm and the later development of lymphoedema in ten patients who had undergone treatment for breast cancer. A more recent study by Clark et al. (2005) of 251 women who had received surgical treatment for breast cancer found that skin puncture performed on the 'at-risk' arm increased the risk of lymphoedema. Damage to an already compromised lymphatic system following surgery may be worsened by the use of a tourniquet to facilitate venous access or initiate an inflammatory response during cannulation which can trigger lymphoedema to develop.
- *Infection.* Postoperative infection of the wound following surgery can add to the damage already sustained by the lymphatic channels during

the surgical procedure. Moses et al. (1982) suggest that infection, developing for any reason, is an overriding factor in the development of lymphoedema. Infection leads to inflammation and an increased capillary filtration rate which can lead to the development of lymphoedema. In addition, the infection can lead to the build-up of debris and the development of scar tissue inside the lymphatic vessels.

Patient-related factors

A range of additional factors associated with the development of swelling have been reported by patients and professionals. These include all conditions/situations where trauma or damage may occur to the tissues of the limb and conditions where an increase in lymphatic load may occur. Many of these factors require further research before their risk in the development of lymphoedema can be clearly determined.

Concurrent medical conditions and medications

Concurrent conditions such as kidney or cardiac disease, diabetes mellitus or hypertension may cause an increase in lymphatic load and increase the risk of lymphoedema developing, but the evidence base to support this rests on physiological assumption only. Chronic conditions such as arthritis, psoriasis and dermatitis cause inflammatory changes to occur within the skin lymphatics. These then become obstructed with debris from the inflammatory process, placing the individual at risk of the development of lymphoedema.

The risk of lymphoedema can also increase when the patient has co-existent venous disease in an 'at-risk' leg. Keeley (2000) suggests that this is because the excess tissue fluid impedes venous return and aggravates the underlying risk of lymphoedema. Patients who are immobile for any reason are also at increased risk of the development of lymphoedema as lymphatic and venous flow is dependent upon muscular activity for efficient function.

There are several medications known to cause fluid retention in some patients for whom they are prescribed. Although there is no firm evidence to indicate whether the risk of lymphoedema may increase as a result of taking these medications, the person at risk of swelling should be made aware of the possible association.

Demographic issues

- *Age*. Lymphoedema is not age specific and can develop after treatment for a wide range of cancers, in addition to the non-cancer related causes previously mentioned. Studies of the incidence of lymphoedema have focused primarily on patients with breast cancer-related swelling and some consider age as a risk factor for the development of lymphoedema within this group.

Segerstrom et al. (1992), in a study of 136 patients treated for breast cancer, did not find a correlation between age and the incidence of lymphoedema, whilst Geller et al. (2003), in a study of 145 women following breast cancer treatment, suggested that there was an increased risk of arm swelling if women were under 50 years of age. Armer & Mei (2005), in a study of 102 women treated for breast cancer, suggested that younger women may have an increased risk of lymphoedema and that this group reported symptoms indicative of lymphoedema more frequently. The symptoms reported by these patients, of arm tenderness, aching and numbness, can be experienced prior to the development of measurable lymphoedema and Armer & Mei (2005) suggest that younger women are less likely to accept these symptoms when they occur, whilst older women are more accepting and consider them as part of the chronic illness process.

As successful management of lymphoedema is dependent upon early identification and management of the condition, it is important that patients of all ages are aware of the early symptoms of lymphoedema and are encouraged to seek help for them if they develop.

- *Weight*. Weight gain and an increased body mass index (BMI) have been considered by some authors as risk factors for the development of lymphoedema. Petrek et al. (2001), in a study of 923 women treated for breast cancer, found a positive correlation between an increased BMI at the time of diagnosis and the development of lymphoedema. The study also found that weight gain in the years following treatment was associated with the development of lymphoedema. In a randomised controlled trial of patients with lymphoedema, Shaw (2004) found that patients randomised to a weight reduction group showed a statistically significant reduction in their arm volume compared to the control group.

  Weight gain and increased BMI are highlighted in other studies which consider the risks of lymphoedema (Hinrichs et al. 2004, Segerstrom et al. 1992) and are not correlated with arm swelling. Geller et al. (2003) suggest that the association with weight gain and lymphoedema requires further investigation due to conflicting results.
- *Use of the limb*. Excessive use of the limb, or exercises which cause increased capillary filtration, can add to the lymph load of the limb. The amount of exercise possible and its intensity will vary between individuals and patients often require advice concerning effective and safe exercises designed to enhance lymph flow, but minimise the risk of

lymphoedema development. Box (2004) supports the maintenance of regular physical activity, suggesting that it promotes lymph drainage and may minimise the risk of lymphoedema developing.

Harris & Niesen-Vertommen (2000) challenged the advice given to patients following axillary surgery to minimise exertive use of the limb and reported the effect of vigorous, repetitive exercise sustained during dragon boat racing on 20 women who were at risk of the development of arm swelling following breast cancer treatment. The study suggests that women may be able to engage in strenuous, repetitive exercise safely without developing lymphoedema, but further research in this area is required.

- *Air travel*. Casley-Smith (1996) suggested that air travel may increase the risk of lymphoedema following breast cancer treatment due to a reduction in barometric pressure. A more recent study by Graham (2002) of 287 women treated for breast cancer concluded that there was no significant difference in the development of lymphoedema between those who had flown and those who had not and that air travel of a domestic or international nature was not a serious hazard to women at risk of lymphoedema. In a three-year follow-up study of patients following breast cancer treatment, Clark et al. (2005) stated that there does not appear to be any firm evidence to support the suggestion that air travel may precipitate swelling in an 'at-risk' limb.

With a lack of clear evidence to balance the risk of lymphoedema development during air travel, it is important that patients are aware of how to look after their 'at-risk' limb prior to, during and after air travel. See Chapter 11 for more information.

Skin conditions

The disruption of lymphatic function that occurs following treatment for cancer involving lymph node areas leads to reduced autoimmune surveillance in the area and an increased risk of infection. Over time, the subcutaneous tissues of the limb can become damaged due to poor lymphatic drainage and fibrosis develops as the lymph fluid pools in the tissues.

Where skin integrity is compromised in patients at risk of lymphoedema, there is a risk of infection entering through broken areas of skin. Dry, flaky skin and superficial fungal infections provide ideal entry points for infection which, once developed, can pose a significant risk of lymphoedema for the patient. Conditions such as psoriasis, eczema and dermatitis also cause an inflammatory response and can initiate the development of lymphoedema unless the condition is controlled.

Trauma sustained by the 'at-risk' limb will initiate an inflammatory response which adds to the fluid load of the limb. The acute swelling that appears following trauma such as sprains and strains is a normal reaction of the body, but may take longer to resolve when lymph drainage in the area is reduced.

The following case scenarios illustrate the history of two different patients who are at risk of the development of lymphoedema.

Case Scenario 1

Karen is a 56-year-old married woman who is recovering from surgery for breast cancer. She underwent the removal of a lump in her right breast and a wide excision of the surrounding tissue. The surgeons also removed eight lymph glands from her axilla to determine the status of her cancer.

Karen recovered well from the surgery, but the wound drainage from her axilla took a long time to reduce and the doctors would not let her go home until the drainage was less than 100 ml in 24 hours. Karen became anxious to go home because she had a family wedding in Scotland and planned to fly to Scotland two days before the wedding so that she could help her sister with the arrangements and spend some time with her niece before her wedding.

Six days after the surgery and five days before the wedding, the wound drain was finally removed, having drained 80 ml over the previous 24 hours. Karen returned to the ward two days later with a small seroma under her axillary scar which required aspiration and on her return from Scotland a week later, more fluid was aspirated before the area settled down.

Consider Karen's history and reflect upon the surgery she has had.

- What risk factors can you identify for the development of lymphoedema in Karen's arm?
- What is the likelihood of Karen developing lymphoedema?

As Karen has had lymph nodes removed from her axilla, the lymphatic drainage will be altered, placing her at risk of the development of lymphoedema. It is estimated that up to one-third of women develop arm swelling following treatment for breast cancer. If lymphoedema does develop it will be because of the surgery and could develop at any time within her lifetime. Karen may be at increased risk of the development of lymphoedema because of the prolonged drainage from her axillary wound and the seroma that formed.

Case Scenario 2

Sean is a 25-year-old student who began travelling overseas with his girlfriend Clare two months ago. They sold their house prior to leaving and planned to travel for two years. A few days before leaving, Sean developed a sore area in his left axilla and noticed a small lump there. He thought it may be due to the fact that he had been busy getting ready to go away and was not really concerned.

Sean and Clare flew to Spain where they bought a vehicle in which they could travel through Europe. A few weeks later the lump in Sean's axilla was bigger and it began to feel painful all the time. He started to take painkillers but when he noticed that his hand and arm were swollen, he went to the hospital for some advice. A biopsy of the lump was taken and Sean was shocked to be told that the lump was due to cancer. He returned home and further tests showed that he had an aggressive form of lymphoma. He commenced chemotherapy and was told that he needed several courses of treatment.

- What risk factors can you identify for the development of lymphoedema in Sean's hand and arm?
- Consider what factors may influence Sean's lymphoedema.

Sean has developed lymphoedema in his arm because of a tumour in the lymph nodes of his axilla. As it has grown, it has obstructed the lymphatic drainage, causing swelling to appear in the hand and arm. The chemotherapy treatment aims to reduce the size of the tumour and as this happens, the lymphatic drainage from the arm should improve, with a noticeable reduction in the swelling.

Sean does not have any identifiable long-term risk factors for lymphoedema because he has not received any surgery or radiotherapy to his axilla. If his cancer is successfully treated, the lymphoedema will resolve but if tumour remains in the axilla or recurs in the future, obstruction of the lymph drainage will cause further swelling.

Conclusion

The number of patients with lymphoedema is unclear and it is thought that many more are at risk of its development through the effects of cancer and its treatment. The presence or occurrence of a wide variety of factors is thought to increase the risk of lymphoedema. However, the identification of those at risk of the development of lymphoedema, regardless of its cause, followed by high-quality, appropriate and timely education may reduce the risk of lymphoedema.

References

Armer J. and Mei R. (2005) Age differences in post-breast cancer lymphoedema signs and symptoms. *Cancer Nursing*, **28**(3): 200–7.

Box R. (2004) Exercise and lymphoedema. *Swell News. Lymphoedema Association of Victoria*, **57**: 1–7.

Casley-Smith J. (1996) Lymphoedema initiated by aircraft flights. *Aviation Space and Environmental Medicine*, **67**(1): 52–6.

Clark B., Sitzia J. and Harlow W. (2005) Incidence and risk of arm oedema following treatment for breast cancer; a three year follow-up study. *Quarterly Journal of Medicine*, **98**(5): 343–8.

Compton L. (1997) A retrospective analysis of 196 patients at a large cancer centre to identify if seroma following axillary dissection is a risk factor for lymphoedema. Unpublished MSc thesis, University of London.

Geller B., Vacek P., O'Brien P. and Secker-Walker R. (2003) Factors associated with arm swelling after breast cancer surgery. *Journal of Women's Health (Larchmt)*, **12**(9): 921–30.

Golshan M., Martin W. and Dowlatshahi K. (2003) Sentinel lymph node biopsy lowers the rate of lymphoedema when compared with standard axillary lymph node dissection. *American Surgery*, **69**(3): 209–11.

Graham P. (2002) Compression prophylaxis may increase the potential for flight-associated lymphoedema after breast cancer treatment. *The Breast*, **11**(1): 66–71.

Hardy D. and Taylor J. (1999) An audit of non-cancer related lymphoedema in a hospice setting. *International Journal of Palliative Nursing*, **5**(1): 18–27.

Harris S. and Niesen-Vertommen S. (2000) Challenging the myth of exercise induced lymphoedema following breast cancer: a series of case reports. *Journal of Surgical Oncology*, **74**(2): 95–9.

Herd-Smith A., Russo A., Muraca M., Del Turco M. and Cardons G. (2001) Prognostic factors for lymphoedema after primary treatment of breast carcinoma. *Cancer*, **92**(7): 1783–7.

Hinrichs C., Watroba N., Rezaishiraz H. et al. (2004) Lymphoedema secondary to postmastectomy radiation: incidence and risk factors. *Annals of Surgical Oncology*, **11**(6): 573–80.

Keeley V. (2000) Classification of lymphoedema. In: R. Twycross, K. Jenns and J. Todd (eds) *Lymphoedema*. Radcliffe Medical Press, Oxford, pp. 22–43.

Kissin M.W., Querci della Rovere Q.G., Easton D. and Westbury G. (1986) Risk of lymphoedema following the treatment of breast cancer. *British Journal of Surgery*, **73**: 580–4.

Kwan W., Jackson J., Weir L., Dingee C., McGregor G. and Olivotto I. (2002) Chronic arm morbidity after curative breast cancer treatment: prevalence and impact on quality of life. *Journal of Clinical Oncology*, **20**(20): 4242–8.

Moses M., Papa M., Karasik A., Reshef A. and Adar R. (1982) The role of infection in post-mastectomy lymphoedema. *Annals of Surgery*, **14**: 73–83.

Mortimer P.S., Bates D.O., Brassington H.D., Stanton A.W.B., Strachan D.P. and Levick J.R. (1996) The prevalence of arm oedema following treatment of breast cancer. *Quarterly Journal of Medicine*, **89**(5): 377–80.

Ottensen E., Duke B. and Karam M. (1997) Strategies and tools for the control/ elimination of lymphatic filariasis. *Bulletin of the World Health Organisation*, **75**(6): 491–503.

Petrek J., Senie R., Peters M. and Rosen P. (2001) Lymphoedema in a cohort of breast carcinoma survivors 20 years after diagnosis. *Cancer*, **92**(6): 1368–77.

Pressman P. (1998) Surgical treatment and lymphoedema. *Cancer*, **83**(S12B): 2782–7.

Querci della Rovere G., Ahmad I., Singe P., Ashley S., Daniels I. and Mortimer P. (2003) An audit of the incidence of arm lymphoedema after prophylactic level 1/11 axillary dissection without division of the pectoralis minor muscle. *Annals of Royal College of Surgeons of England*, **85**(3): 1–4.

Ryan M., Stainton M., Slaytor E., Jaconelli C., Watts S. and Mackenzie P. (2003) Aetiology and prevalence of lower limb lymphoedema following treatment for gynaecological cancer. *Australia and New Zealand Journal of Obstetrics and Gynaecology*, **43**(2): 148–51.

Segerstrom K., Bjerle P., Graffmas S. and Nystrom A. (1992) Factors which influence the incidence of brachial oedema after treatment of breast cancer. *Scandinavian Journal of Plastic and Reconstructive Surgery and Hand Surgery*, **26**(2): 223–7.

Sener S., Winchester D., Martz C. et al. (2001) Lymphedema after sentinel lymphadenectomy for breast carcinoma. *Cancer*, **92**(4): 748–52.

Shaw C. (2004) *Dietary Interventions: lymphoedema, diet and body weight in breast cancer patients*. Annual Research Report. Royal Marsden NHS Foundation Trust and Institute of Cancer Research, London, pp. 58–61.

Sitzia J., Woods M., Hine P., Williams A., Eaton K. and Green G. (1998) Characteristics of new referrals to twenty seven lymphoedema treatment units. *European Journal of Cancer Care*, **7**(4): 255–62.

Smith J. (1998) The practice of venepuncture in lymphoedema. *European Journal of Cancer Care*, **7**(2): 97–8.

Stanton A., Levick J. and Mortimer P. (1996) Current puzzles presented by post-mastectomy oedema (breast cancer related lymphoedema). *Vascular Medicine*, **1**: 213–25.

Tadych K. and Donegan W. (1987) Post-mastectomy seromas and wound drainage. *Surgery, Gynaecology and Obstetrics*, **165**: 483–7.

Werngren-Elgstrom M. and Lidman D. (1994) Lymphoedema of the lower extremities after surgery and radiotherapy for cancer of the cervix. *Scandinavian Journal of Plastic and Reconstructive Surgery and Hand Surgery*, **28**(4): 289–93.

Williams A., Franks P. and Moffatt C. (2005) Lymphoedema: estimating the size of the problem. *Palliative Medicine*, **19**(4): 300–13.

World Health Organisation (1998) *Measuring Health. World Health Report. Life in the 21st Century: a vision for all*. World Health Organisation, Geneva, pp. 45–67.

3 Educating the Patient at Risk of Lymphoedema

Introduction

The development of lymphoedema cannot be prevented but the risks associated with its appearance can be minimised by the adoption of precautions which avoid overloading the remaining lymphatics. Those at risk of developing lymphoedema should be advised concerning these precautions by health-care professionals who can establish why the patient may develop lymphoedema and identify their education needs.

The aim of this chapter is to prepare the health-care professional for a role that includes educating the patient at risk of the development of lymphoedema and enabling them to provide such patients with knowledge to promote positive health behaviours in the care of their 'at-risk' limb.

Learning objectives

At the end of this chapter the reader will be able to:

- outline the educational needs of the patient who is at risk of the development of lymphoedema
- describe precautions that can be taken to minimise the risk of lymphoedema developing
- discuss relevant sources of advice and information on lymphoedema for patients and professionals.

Educational needs

Any disruption to the lymphatic system caused by cancer or its treatment will place a patient at risk of the development of lymphoedema. Education

concerning this risk should commence when consent is gained for any treatment which may compromise lymphatic function, so that the patient is fully
aware of the implications. This is often a difficult time, when a new diagnosis is being faced and decisions are being made about treatment, but it is
essential that information concerning all potential side effects to treatment
are included to ensure that the patient is fully informed.

Lymphatic intervention as a part of cancer treatment cannot always be
avoided and in circumstances where it is necessary, the patient should
receive appropriate information and long-term advice to enable them to
care for their 'at-risk' limb and minimise the risk of lymphoedema developing. All verbal advice should be appropriate and timely, culturally sensitive
and supported by written information. Several cancer charities and patient
support groups, listed at the end of this book, provide written information
for patients concerning lymphoedema.

The British Lymphology Society (2001) stated that patients at risk of lymphoedema should receive advice about:

- why they are at risk
- the implications of being at risk
- what they can do to minimise the risk of developing lymphoedema
- what action they should take if swelling develops.

Morgan et al. (2005), in a study of 54 community nurses' level of knowledge
of lymphoedema, found that the nurses understood their role in educating
patients about lymphoedema and offering appropriate advice, but lacked
a knowledge base to enable them to fulfil this role. Knowledge of the
risks associated with lymphoedema was perceived as 'poor' by 30 of the
study group. The nurses considered that the patients' general practitioners
viewed their roles differently and rather than educating patients, perceived
their role primarily as providing intervention when clinically indicated.

The lack of understanding of the professional roles in providing advice and
care for this group of patients, Morgan et al. (2005) believe, has led to a perception that lymphoedema is a low-priority problem. It is clear that if patients
are to receive the advice they require from health-care professionals at all
levels, educational programmes should be provided to prepare them ade-
quately and if patients are to minimise their risk of developing lymphoedema, their long-term care is the responsibility of all health-care professionals.

Precautions to minimise the risk of lymphoedema

Once a risk of lymphoedema development has been established, education
and advice should focus on minimising the risk by reducing strain on the
lymphatic system. Much of the patient literature available provides a list of

'do's and don'ts' for patients to follow. This advice should be supported with a clear explanation of the rationale behind it.

Avoiding infection

The immunological response of the body is dependent upon an efficient lymph system and those at risk of lymphoedema through a disruption to lymph flow will have an altered immune surveillance (Linnett 2000). If a bacterial infection enters through a break in the skin to involve the superficial layers of the skin and subcutaneous tissues when lymph drainage is reduced, the inflammatory response that results will increase the lymphatic load and may precipitate the onset of lymphoedema.

It is therefore essential that the skin of the 'at-risk' limb is kept clean, healthy and intact. Table 3.1 outlines recommended actions that the patient should adopt in daily life in order to minimise the risk of infection in an 'at-risk' limb and the rationale for the actions outlined.

Encouraging lymph drainage

Surgery or radiotherapy to lymph node areas causes an alteration in the transport capacity of the remaining lymph channels. The lymph load has to drain through narrower channels and the lymph pump can easily become overloaded. If excess lymph fluid is produced, the transport capacity of the remaining lymphatics can become overwhelmed, with the result that swelling appears in the limb. By avoiding activities where the lymph load may increase, drainage from the limb can be maintained and the risk of lymphoedema minimised.

Table 3.2 outlines recommended actions that the patient should follow to promote lymph drainage.

Considering everyday activities

The risk of developing lymphoedema can be decreased by the moderation of activities which may bring more blood into the area and therefore increase the lymph load. Patients should be advised regarding specific exercises, activities and hobbies, but the principle to follow is that activities of an exertive, strenuous nature should be avoided and gentler activities aimed at promoting lymph drainage encouraged.

Table 3.3 highlights some activities that the patient at risk of lymphoedema may have to consider.

Table 3.1   Care of the skin to avoid infection.

Action to follow	Rationale
Wash the skin daily with soap and dry carefully.	To promote skin hygiene.
Keep the skin moist and well hydrated by using a moisturising cream daily.	To prevent skin dryness and chafing and promote skin integrity.
Treat any cuts or breaks in the skin antiseptically.	To minimise the risk of infection.
Use a high-factor suncream if the skin is exposed to the sun or cover the affected area.	Sunburn causes an inflammatory response and increased lymphatic load as the body tries to correct the damage to the skin.
Use an insect repellent if there is a likelihood of mosquito bites.	The piercing of the skin and the vector of the mosquito are risk factors for infection.
If the arm is at risk, wear protective gloves when using the oven, using household cleaning agents and gardening.	To minimise the risk of accidental trauma to the skin which can lead to infection.
Use an electric razor rather than a blade razor or chemical hair remover when removing unwanted body hair.	To avoid trauma and damage to the skin.
Avoid needle sticks, blood tests, injections and intravenous infusions in the limb that is at risk.	Lymphoedema may be triggered by an inflammatory response to the skin puncture or the development of infection entering through the skin.
Pay attention to care of the nails on the hands or feet: do not cut or tear cuticles – use a cuticle stick covered with cotton wool.	To avoid trauma to the skin which may result in infection.
Wear well-fitting, comfortable shoes if the feet are affected.	To prevent trauma to the skin and the formation of blisters which may cause infection.

Sources of education and advice

Patients

Individual needs vary regarding the type, amount and timing of support, information and advice. It is important that the health-care professional is

Table 3.2 Activities to encourage lymph drainage.

Action to follow	Rationale
Avoid chemical hair removers when removing unwanted hair.	These can irritate the skin, causing an inflammatory response and increased lymphatic load which may result in lymphoedema.
Avoid extremes of temperature such as hot baths and cold showers.	Sudden changes of temperature in the limb can cause an increase in lymph load and the development of lymphoedema.
If the arm is at risk, offer the other unaffected arm when blood pressure recordings are required.	To avoid constriction of the lymphatic channels.
Wear loose clothing that does not constrict the limb.	The remaining lymphatics need to be allowed to drain freely.
Make sure that any jewellery does not constrict the limb.	Tight jewellery may constrict lymph channels and any indentation of the skin may lead to inflammation and increased lymph load.
Follow an exercise regime of gentle, regular exercise such as swimming, walking or yoga which does not overexert the affected limb.	Lymph drainage is promoted by regular muscular activity.

Table 3.3 Reducing the risk of lymphoedema to promote lymph drainage.

Action to follow	Rationale
Avoid strenuous activities with the affected limb such as pushing, pulling, carrying and lifting activities; carry or lift light loads only.	These activities can cause a strain on the muscles of the limb and lead to inflammation and an increased lymph load.
Avoid repetitive movements with the affected limb, especially those against resistance.	Repetitive movements can increase the lymph load.
If the leg is affected, wear well-fitting shoes or sandals at all times.	To protect the feet from injury or trauma.
If the leg is affected, try to avoid standing in one position for long periods.	Lymph drainage can be reduced if the muscles become inactive.
Keep body weight within normal limits by eating a healthy diet.	If excess weight is carried, more strain can be put on the compromised lymph load.
It is important to rest if the affected limb begins to ache, feel tired or heavy.	Overexertion will cause the limb to become tired and additional lymph fluid to be produced which will take time to drain.

sensitive to the patient's needs and verbal information should always be supported with written information that can be referred to at a later date. Many patients will source further information via the internet where a wealth of advice is available. As this is not regulated, it is important that patients are given the opportunity to discuss any information they acquire with a health-care professional to ensure that it is relevant to them.

Details of patient-focused publications available from cancer charities and additional internet-based sources, both national and international, can be found at the back of this book.

Health-care professionals

Health-care professionals with an interest in lymphoedema can find support, information and professional activities via the British Lymphology Society which is a multidisciplinary organisation open to all health-care professionals. Many compression therapy companies also offer educational support to health-care professionals. Contact details are presented at the back of this book.

The following case scenario outlines the educational needs of a patient who is at risk of the development of lymphoedema of the leg.

Case Scenario

Ian is a 52-year-old married man with two teenage children aged 16 years and 18 years, who works as an accountant. Several months ago he noticed a lump in his right thigh which he initially ignored, thinking it was a tennis injury or a bruise. When it persisted, his doctor referred him for a biopsy and Ian was shocked to find out the lump was a sarcoma. He underwent excision of the lump and the removal of lymph nodes in his groin.

Ian is very distressed about his diagnosis. His sister died a year ago from breast cancer and he found this an extremely upsetting time. He was close to his sister and had not experienced someone with cancer before. His family are also shocked by his diagnosis and concerned about the implications. Ian is normally an active man who plays tennis regularly and shares a love of music with his wife. He works primarily from home, but his work requires a commitment to long hours and he sometimes works late at night or during the weekend to meet deadlines. His wife is very supportive, but also works full time in a demanding job and wonders if she should try to arrange to be at home more now for her husband.

Ian recovered well from the surgery although he developed some swelling in his leg immediately after the operation. Before he was discharged home he was told that lymphoedema may develop in the future because the lymph nodes had been removed.

Consider Ian's diagnosis and recent treatment.

- What information would you give him about his risk of developing lymphoedema?
- Consider what you know of his lifestyle and home situation and outline the main priorities in the advice he requires in caring for his leg.

Ian is at risk of developing lymphoedema because of the surgery to the lymph nodes in his groin. He is trying to come to terms with his diagnosis and therefore will only be able to absorb limited information initially. However, it is important that he and his wife are made aware of the risk of lymphoedema and that all verbal information given is supported with written information which he can refer to later.

1. Why he is at risk of lymphoedema

The surgery to the lymph nodes in his groin will influence the drainage of lymph from the leg to this area. The lymph drainage system can be likened to a motorway: when there are roadworks on the motorway, the traffic has to slow down and use a reduced number of traffic lanes. Some traffic will exit the motorway early to avoid the congestion and the rest will exit as normal but find that their journey takes longer.

2. The implications of being at risk

The lymph nodes play a major role in the surveillance and fighting of infection. Because there are a reduced number of lymph nodes in the groin, there is an increased risk of infection in the adjacent leg because the lymph fluid takes longer to drain away.

3. What Ian can do to minimise the risk of lymphoedema developing

- His regular physical activity is good and should be recommenced as soon as he is able as it will promote lymph drainage. Ian should listen to his body, though, and if his leg aches or feels sore, he may need to modify his activity and do a little less or play tennis for shorter periods of time.
- He should consider his work activities and avoid sitting or standing for long periods as these will discourage lymph from draining. Regular breaks from work to stretch his legs and move around are a good idea. He could support his legs on a stool whilst working to encourage lymph drainage.
- He should protect his legs from cuts or breaks by ensuring his shoes fit well, keep his leg clean and ensure he is protected from sunburn and mosquito bites when he goes on holiday.

- He should ensure that any cuts or breaks sustained to the skin are treated with antiseptic cream as soon as possible, to minimise the risk of infection, and take good care of his skin at all times.

4.   Action to take if swelling develops in his leg

- Ian should be advised that the swelling that developed in his leg after surgery is of an acute nature and should settle over the next few days.
- If he notices prolonged swelling, he should seek advice from his hospital consultant or general practitioner.
- The risk of lymphoedema is lifelong so if swelling develops at any time in the future, advice should be sought from his hospital consultant or general practitioner.
- Details of a health-care professional or organisation that he can contact for further advice about lymphoedema should be provided.

Conclusion

Educating the patient at risk of lymphoedema should start as early as possible and ideally, before the procedure that is likely to impact on lymph drainage takes place. There is evidence to suggest that incorporating some simple, positive health behaviours into normal daily patterns can help to minimise the risk of lymphoedema. Precautions to follow should include activities to avoid infection and encourage lymph drainage in the affected limb.

References

British Lymphology Society (2001) *Chronic Oedema Population and Needs*. British Lymphology Society, Surrey. Available at: www.lymphoedema.org/bls (accessed 21/10/05).

Linnett N. (2000) Skin management in lymphoedema. In: R. Twycross, K. Jenns and J. Todd (eds) *Lymphoedema*. Radcliffe Medical Press, Oxford, pp. 118–29.

Morgan P., Moody M., Franks P., Moffatt C. and Doherty D. (2005) Assessing community nurses; level of knowledge of lymphoedema. *British Journal of Nursing*, **14**(1): 8–13.

4 Identifying Secondary Lymphoedema

Introduction

The appearance of secondary lymphoedema is rarely a sudden event. The swelling usually develops over a period of time as the transport capacity of the lymphatic channels becomes unable to meet the demands of the lymphatic load. Early, uncomplicated lymphoedema differs from advanced lymphoedema in which characteristic clinical features can be observed due to the stasis of lymph fluid causing progressive changes in the subcutaneous tissues and skin.

Lymphoedema can affect the head and neck, limbs, breast, trunk or genitalia depending upon the area where lymph drainage has been interrupted. In some cases a limb and its adjacent truncal quadrant are involved in the swelling. The diagnosis of lymphoedema should always be based on a subjective and objective observation combined with a clinical history in which relevant risk factors for the development of swelling are identified.

The aim of this chapter is to assist the health-care professional in identifying lymphoedema by considering relevant factors in its appearance and development. Methods of limb assessment will then be considered in order to prepare the health-care professional for their role in advising the patient concerning the management of mild, uncomplicated lymphoedema.

Learning objectives

At the end of this chapter the reader will be able to:

- outline a staging model for lymphoedema based on clinical features
- discuss the clinical features associated with lymphoedema
- describe how measurements of a limb can be made and when they are indicated.

Table 4.1   International Society of Lymphology (2000) staging of lymphoedema.

Stage 1	<ul><li>Tissues are soft with no fibrosis</li><li>Oedema pits on pressure and reduces with limb elevation</li><li>Limb volume difference <20%</li></ul>
Stage 2	<ul><li>Substantial fibrosis</li><li>Tissues feel firm</li><li>Oedema does not pit on pressure or reduce on elevation</li><li>Risk of infection is increased</li><li>Limb volume difference >20%</li></ul>
Stage 3	<ul><li>Severe skin changes: hyperkeratosis and papillomatosis</li><li>Skin loses elasticity</li><li>Skin folds develop</li><li>Risk of infection increases</li><li>Limb volume difference >40%</li></ul>

Stages in the development of secondary lymphoedema

The staging of any disease can be helpful in order to identify the extent of the problem so that realistic treatment decisions and management plans can be made. Two models of lymphoedema staging have been described, the first by the International Society of Lymphology (ISL) (2000) and the second by the British Lymphology Society (BLS) (2001).

- The ISL model (2000) outlined in Table 4.1 describes a three-stage developmental process in which lymphoedema is classified according to physical signs associated with the appearance of swelling. Consideration is not given to any psychosocial and psychological aspects of the lymphoedema.
- The BLS model (2001) outlined in Table 4.2 also considers the severity of a patient's lymphoedema according to physical symptoms and outlines four categories within which patients can be considered. The model includes consideration of quality of life issues where more severe, complex oedema is present and also acknowledges the needs of patients at risk of the development of lymphoedema.

Whilst a staging system can be useful in the identification of lymphoedema and to reflect improvements over time, it is important to remember that many patients will not fit neatly into the categories outlined and such systems can therefore be restrictive.

In the period immediately following surgery involving the lymphatic channels, acute swelling may occur, which is usually transient and mild, developing as a result of the trauma to the lymphatic channels. A further type of acute lymphoedema may develop 6–8 weeks postoperatively,

Table 4.2 British Lymphology Society (2001) classification of lymphoedema.

Group 1: People at risk	Group 2: Mild, uncomplicated lymphoedema	Group 3: Moderate to severe/complicated lymphoedema	Group 4: Oedema in advanced disease
Symptoms may include: • No clinical signs of oedema • Risk factors for oedema can be identified	Symptoms may include: • Excess limb volume <20% • No involvement of the trunk, genitals or digits • Intact, healthy skin • Normal limb shape preserved • No venous or arterial complications • No active malignancy	Symptoms may include: • Swelling present in the trunk, digits or genitals • Distorted limb shape • Skin in poor condition • Active or controlled malignancy • Presence of complications, e.g. infection, lymphorrhoea • Moderate lymphoedema: excess limb volume greater than 20% but not more than 40% • Severe lymphoedema: excess limb volume 40% or more	Symptoms may include: • Uncontrolled metastatic disease • Weeping/ulceration of affected limb • Impaired function • Impaired mobility • Impaired sensation • Pain • Infection • Oedema of face, genitals, trunk

possibly as a result of inflammation in the lymphatic drainage routes. This pattern of lymphoedema may be observed during a course of radiation treatment and frequently resolves slowly but spontaneously, with minimal intervention. Acute swelling developing in the immediate or postoperative period is not a known predictor of the development of further chronic swelling.

The patient may then enter a subclinical or latency period, described as Stage 0 by Foldi & Foldi (2003), where swelling is not present although there are risk factors for its development. This stage may exist for many years and never progress any further (Mortimer et al. 1996).

Early-onset lymphoedema may then develop. At this stage, swelling will be noticeable but may be intermittent and transient and related to an exertive or prolonged activity involving the affected limb, or triggered by infection in the limb. If management of this early lymphoedema is not

Table 4.3   Stages of lymphoedema development (adapted from Foldi & Foldi 2003).

Stage	Description	Features
0	Subclinical or latency period	• Regional lymph nodes have been resected and the transport capacity of the lymph system is reduced, but still sufficient to transport the lymph load. • Swelling is NOT present. • This stage may exist for many years.
I	Reversible	• Early-onset lymphoedema due to a decrease in the transport capacity of the lymphatics. • The swollen tissues are soft upon palpation and may swell intermittently only. • Thumb pressure on the tissues causes pitting. • The limb shape is maintained. • The swelling may reduce overnight when at rest or on elevation.
II	Spontaneously irreversible	• The transport capacity of the lymphatic system is unable to meet the demands of the lymph load and tissue changes become evident due to lymph stasis. • The swelling is constant and does not reduce on elevation or at rest. • The tissues become brawny and firm. • Pitting of the tissues on gentle thumb pressure becomes more difficult. • The swelling may affect the limb shape.
III	Elephantiasis	• The stasis of fluid and protein leads to chronic fibrosis of the connective tissue and an increased risk of infection from impaired lymph clearance. • The tissues are hard and fibrotic. • Pitting of the tissues is absent. • The skin becomes thickened. Warty overgrowths become evident and hyperpigmentation is evident. • The limb can swell to enormous proportions, lose its shape and develop skin folds and creases.

commenced, the swelling may progress to become permanently present and eventually the skin and tissues will begin to undergo changes from the stasis of lymph fluid.

The development of chronic lymphoedema is indicated by characteristic changes occurring in the tissues and skin. Table 4.3 outlines the stages of lymphoedema development and the tissue and skin changes that are characteristic of each stage as described by Foldi & Foldi (2003).

Clinical features

A range of clinical features are used to identify lymphoedema and their presence and severity can help to indicate which type of management is required in order to control the swelling.

Oedema

Quade (2004) suggested that oedema is not clinically detectable until the interstitial fluid volume is 30% above normal. Oedema may be visible in part or all of a limb. If the affected limb is compared to the contralateral limb, it is possible to establish the visible distribution of the swelling. Oedema may also develop in the adjacent truncal quadrant. Figure 4.1 illustrates secondary lymphoedema of the leg.

Lymphoedema usually develops over a period of time to a point when it becomes noticeable by the patient. This time of onset may be associated with a particular event or activity and this can provide information upon which patient education can be focused in order to prevent a worsening of the condition. A dominant arm may be bigger than a non-dominant arm due to the additional activities it is subjected to, particularly if these are strenuous, and these factors will need to be considered in any observation for the presence of lymphoedema.

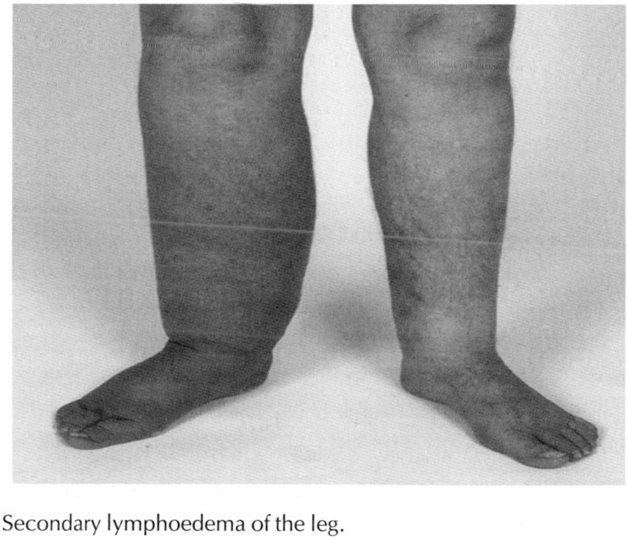

Figure 4.1   Secondary lymphoedema of the leg.

Tissue changes

The subcutaneous tissues usually have a soft, doughy consistency when lifted or palpated. If lymphoedema is present, light thumb or finger pressure on the tissues results in an indentation or pitting as the fluid is displaced. As the condition progresses the tissues harden due to the fibrotic changes. At this stage fluid can no longer be displaced and pitting becomes more difficult.

A highly specific test for lymphoedema, Stemmer's sign, is considered indicative of whether swelling is present (Board & Harlow 2002, Keeley 2000). A positive Stemmer's sign is thickened skin at the base of the second toe due to the stasis of lymph fluid which results in an inability to pick up a fold of skin.

Skin changes

The skin remains a normal colour when swelling is present and any alteration in colour should be medically investigated to exclude problematic complications such as infection, venous thrombosis or active disease.

A variety of skin changes may be visible depending upon the degree of swelling present and its duration.

- Dry skin
- Shiny or taut skin
- Skin folds and crevices

As lymphoedema progresses, further changes occur in the skin and the following may become evident.

- Infection: the limb is hot, red and tender
- Lymphorrhoea: leakage of lymph fluid from the skin
- Hyperkeratosis: the skin is warty and scaly as a result of long-term swelling
- Papillomatosis: a cobblestone appearance on the skin due to dilated skin lymphatics
- Lymphangiomas: lymph blisters giving the appearance of frogspawn.

Further information about skin conditions can be found in Chapter 6 and complications of lymphoedema can be found in Chapter 12.

Pain and discomfort

Lymphoedema is not normally painful but discomfort of varying degrees is often reported by patients. During the initial stages in the development of swelling, a tension in the tissues or tightening in the skin may be experienced. Though this is uncomfortable, it should not be painful and should not cause any functional impairment.

When the swelling is more advanced, sensations of aching and heaviness within the limb may be experienced. There may be some functional impairment at this stage as the weight of the swollen limb and degree of swelling begin to restrict movement. A heavy, swollen arm can cause problems with shoulder mobility and a heavy swollen leg can lead to back and hip problems.

Altered sensations, such as tingling, numbness and burning in the limb, can sometimes be experienced and these symptoms require further medical investigation.

Psychological and psychosocial problems

The development of lymphoedema can have a negative impact on many areas of the patient's life. A physical alteration in the appearance of the body can cause problems with body image which for some patients are difficult to reconcile. Physical difficulties can result in emotions of anger, anxiety and depression whilst relationships can suffer and present the potential for isolation and withdrawal (see Chapter 5).

Measuring lymphoedema

Stanton et al. (1996) suggest that swelling of an area of the body is usually observed by the patient first. This view is supported in a study by Clark et al. (2005) in which women who developed arm swelling were reported to have observed the swelling themselves and then actively sought advice regarding its management. Where one limb is involved, a visible comparison with the contralateral, normal limb can provide an indication of any alteration in limb shape or size.

Various non-invasive methods of measuring limbs can then provide further information concerning the distribution of any swelling. Measurements of the limb can also assist in decisions regarding the need for further advice and management of the swelling or referral to a more experienced practitioner. Measurement of swelling in other areas of the body such as the head and neck, the trunk or the breast is more difficult and subjective assessment is utilised instead of a standard measurement technique.

When is swelling present?

Natural differences in size occur between healthy dominant and non-dominant arms and also between healthy left and right legs (Stanton et al.

Table 4.4   Measurement approaches used to identify lymphoedema.

Method	Advantages	Disadvantages
Water displacement *The oldest recorded method of measuring the difference between limbs*	• Easy to measure lower limbs • Can accurately measure the volume of the feet or hands	• Patient needs to be agile • Distribution of oedema is not indicated • Temperature of the water needs to be appropriate • Can be a messy procedure if water spillage occurs • It is difficult to submerge arms • There is the potential for cross-infection
Surface measurements *The most frequently used method of measuring limbs today*	• A practical method for objectively measuring limbs • Quick and easy to do with minimal training required	• Accuracy can be influenced by the measurer • The volume of the feet and hands are excluded • Cannot record shape/contour of the limb
Perometry *An opto-electrical imaging system which measures the volume of the limb using light beams*	• Provides data on limb size and shape • Quick and easy to use following training • Not influenced by different operators • Studies have confirmed reliability	• Very expensive • Space required for the positioning of the machine • Not portable
Advanced imagery *(CT, MRI, bio-electrical impedance analyser, ultrasound)*	• Possibly more detailed in information acquired	• Confined space can be claustrophobic • Expensive • Not appropriate for routine use with large numbers of patients

2000). Dominant arms in healthy women were shown by Kettle et al. (1958) to be as much as 3.9% larger than the non-dominant arms and a difference of 2.9% was reported by Katch & Weltman (1975) in a study of the difference between normal legs, which did not account for dominance. A measurable threshold, above which it may be said that swelling is present, has been considered (Armer et al. 2003, Kissin et al. 1986) and where arm swelling is reported, a measurable difference greater than 2 cm at a corresponding point on the contralateral limb or an excess volume of 200 ml is considered symptomatic of lymphoedema. A similar measurable threshold for leg swelling has not been reported.

Measurement of limb size should always be considered in conjunction with observation for the presence of any of the clinical features that have already been discussed in this chapter. In advanced lymphoedema, tissue shrinkage may occur due to extensive fibrosis and in this case measurement of the limb in isolation may be misleading.

Measuring limb size

The measuring of limb size is a useful objective means of determining if swelling is present or if the limb size has changed following a previous measurement. Several techniques have been described, each with advantages and disadvantages. Table 4.4 summarises the different measurement techniques used to measure swelling in a limb.

Surface measurements

The technique most frequently used for measuring limb size involves surface measurements recorded in centimetres of either upper or lower limbs using a plastic-coated tape measure. These can be simple surface measurements or more detailed limb volume measurements taken at regular 4 cm intervals along the length of the limb.

Simple surface measurements
Figures 4.2 and 4.3 illustrate the techniques used to record simple measurements of an arm and a leg.

- Circumference measurements of the swollen and contralateral limb are recorded in centimetres at four identifiable points on each limb and compared.
- The measurements are taken to provide a basic indication of any difference between the contralateral limbs.
- This technique of measuring is frequently used to provide a guide to the selection of compression garments.
- Simple measurements of a limb are a useful means of assessment and evaluation when detailed measurements are not required. This may be because a patient is unwell or has advanced disease.

Equipment required when recording simple surface measurements: skin marker, a narrow plastic-coated tape measure, appropriate documentation to record the measurements clearly.

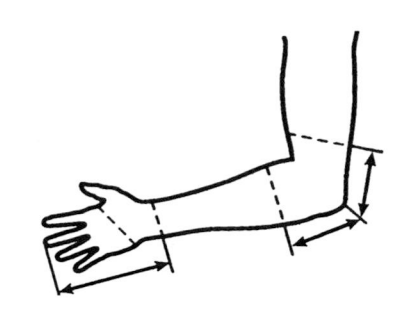

Measure from the tip of the 3rd finger to a place on the wrist where the tape measure will lie flat. Mark and record this point. Measure the circumference of the arm at this point and record in the documentation.

Measure the circumference of the hand at the widest point. Mark the olecranon and make a mark 10 cm below and above this mark. Mark each of these points and measure the circumference of the arm at each point, recording it clearly in the documentation.

Figure 4.2   Simple surface measurements of the arm.

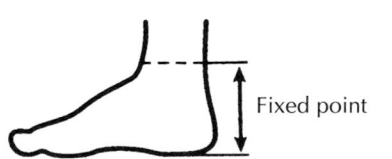

Measure a distance from the base of the heel to a point above the ankle where the tape measure lies flat. Record this distance and mark the position of the point. Measure the circumference of the leg at this point and record in the documentation. Identify the patella and mark a point 15 cm above and 15 cm below. Measure the circumference of the leg at this point and record in the documentation.

Figure 4.3   Simple surface measurements of the leg.

Limb volume measurements

Figures 4.4 and 4.5 illustrate the technique of recording limb volume measurements for the upper limbs and the legs.

● Circumference measurements of the swollen and contralateral limb are recorded in centimetres at 4 cm intervals along the length of the limb.

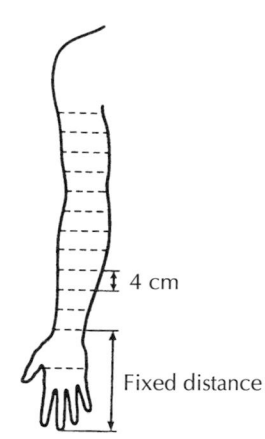

- Ask the patient to relax their arm and position it horizontally, supported on a table or the back of a chair.

- Measure and mark the distance from the tip of the middle finger to the wrist and record the distance accurately. The fixed starting point will be used on each subsequent measuring occasion.

- Mark intervals of 4 cm along the length of the arm using a ruler or tape measure.

- Measure the circumference of the hand at the widest point and record this measurement. It is not used in calculations of limb volume.

- Measure the circumference of the arm at each marked point, ensuring that the arm is straight and that the tape measure lies smoothly on the arm without tension.

Figure 4.4 Limb volume measurement of the arm.

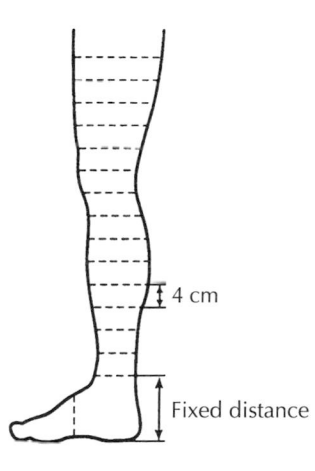

- Ask the patient to relax their leg and position it horizontally, supported on a couch or bed.

- With the foot flexed, measure and mark the distance from the heel to the ankle and record this distance accurately. The fixed starting point will be used on each subsequent measuring occasion.

- Mark intervals of 4 cm along the inner aspect of the leg using a ruler or tape measure.

- Measure the circumference of the foot at the widest point and record this measurement. It is not used in calculations of limb volume.

- Measure the circumference of the leg at each marked point, ensuring that the tape measure lies smoothly on the leg without tension.

Figure 4.5 Limb volume measurement of the leg.

- The limb volume is determined by applying the measurements recorded to the mathematical formula used to calculate the volume of a cylinder.
- This technique of surface measurements taken at 4 cm intervals provides a more detailed image of the distribution of swelling along

Table 4.5   Standardisation of limb volume measurements to ensure reproducibility and accuracy.

Action	Rationale
Mark the limb with new marks each time measurements are taken.	If the limb shape or size has changed, old marks will not be accurately positioned.
Never put tension on the tape measure.	Any tension applied will vary between measurers and result in inconsistent measurements being recorded.
Document the starting point chosen on the limb accurately.	To ensure that the same starting point is used each time measurements are taken.
Use the same number of measurements each time.	To ensure that the same section of the limb is measured each time and enable comparison with other limb volumes to be made.
Measure the limb in a horizontal, resting position.	Tension on the muscles of the limb and fluctuations in the position of the limb during measuring can lead to inaccuracies.
Measure both limbs each time.	To enable a limb volume difference to be calculated.
Do not include the hand or foot measurement in calculations of limb volume.	The mathematical formula used with limb volume measurements calculates the volume of a cylinder and the hand and foot do not form part of a cylinder.
Use the same resting position each time measurements are taken.	The shape and size of the limb are influenced by the degree of flexion or relaxation of the muscles and can therefore influence the measurements taken.

the length of the limb and can illustrate changes in the limb size over time.
- The measurements can be used to determine the excess volume of the swollen limb when compared to the contralateral limb.
- Calculations can be complex and lengthy unless a preprogrammed calculator is used.
- The measurements can be inaccurate unless attention is paid to standardisation of the measuring technique. Table 4.5 outlines considerations to ensure reproducibility and accuracy.

Calculating limb volume

Once all the measurements of the limb have been recorded, the volume of the limb can be determined. The mathematical formula for calculating the

Table 4.6   Calculating total limb volume.

Circumference measurements recorded in cm	Circumference^2 $\overline{\Pi}$ (measurement squared then divided by 3.14 to calculate volume)	Volumes added to calculate total limb volume
18.4	107.8	107.8
19.1	116.2	224.0
21.2	143.1	367.1
23.7	179.0	546.1
24.8	195.9	742.0
25.7	210.2	952.2
26.6	225.2	1177.4
28.8	264.2	1441.6
29.6	278.8	1720.4
30.9	304.1	2024.5
31.7	319.8	2344.3
33.5	357.2	2701.5

Total limb volume = 2701.5 ml

volume of a cylinder is used as it considers the limb as a series of cylinders, each with a height of 4 cm. The formula is:

$$\frac{Circumference^2}{\Pi}$$

By totalling the volumes of all the cylinders, the total limb volume can be reached. Table 4.6 illustrates how total limb volume measurements are calculated. The calculation is lengthy and can be speeded up if a programmable calculator is used with the mathematical formula already programmed in.

If the limb volume of the opposite limb is also calculated, the excess volume in the swollen limb can be estimated. The following is an example of how this can be done.

Swollen left arm limb volume   2701.5 ml
   minus
Normal right arm limb volume   2394.8 ml
   equals   <u>306.7 mls</u>

The swollen left arm is 306 ml larger than the normal right arm. This can now be expressed as a percentage difference:

100 ÷ Normal limb volume × volume difference between the two arms
100 ÷ 2394.8 × 306.7 = 13%

The swollen left arm is 13% bigger than the normal right arm.

When should measurements be recorded?

Patients often place great significance on measurements taken of a limb but the technique is only one method of obtaining valuable information regarding the presence of swelling. The observation of other clinical features such as the condition of the skin, shape of the limb and function of the limb also provides valuable information.

Armer et al. (2003) argue that limb volume measurements should be taken before the patient undergoes any surgery involving lymph node areas, to ensure that a normal baseline measurement is available for comparison should swelling subsequently develop. This view is shared by Piller (1999) who states that such measurements enable changes to be detected more accurately and more cost-effective treatment to be commenced. The recording of simple surface measurements of limbs preoperatively may be a simpler, quicker and more suitable alternative than the more complex limb volume measurements.

When lymphoedema is suspected or reported, limb volume measurements of the affected and contralateral limb should be recorded. These provide a baseline upon which progress can be measured and treatment decisions can be made. In order to evaluate progress, measurements should be repeated every few months, particularly when swelling has been observed and is undergoing active management. Limb volume measurements are completed more frequently during a course of multilayer compression bandaging because the limb size and shape can undergo quite marked changes over a short period of time. Final measurements should be recorded at the end of a course of treatment.

Simple surface measurements provide an alternative means of assessment and evaluation and can be useful if a patient is unwell or has advanced disease and detailed limb volume measurements are not indicated. The measurements also provide a guide for the therapist when choosing the size of compression garments for the patient, although the final size should be determined by the patient's comfort and not the size indicated by the measurements taken.

The following case scenarios are presented to highlight relevant factors in the identification of secondary lymphoedema.

Case Scenario 1

Julia is a 40-year-old mother of two young children, who underwent a left mastectomy and axillary clearance for breast cancer three months ago. She developed some swelling in her arm immediately after the surgery but once she got home and back to normal, she no longer noticed it. Her radiotherapy treatment to the chest wall was completed without any problems, but a few days later Julia noticed that her wedding ring was tight and that her left hand was swollen. She became aware of a feeling of tightness in her left arm and began to get worried. She now thinks that the left sleeve of her clothes feels tight but wonders if she is imagining this.

The family moved house a week ago and Julia has been busy unpacking boxes and moving furniture to create a new home quickly. She wants to get back to normal because the children have been unsettled due to her cancer treatment and the recent house move and she wants them to feel settled and secure again quickly. She is worried that the swelling indicates that she has further problems and is upset at the thought of more treatment.

Julia presents with mild swelling that is visible in her left arm. Her hand is slightly swollen and swelling extends from the wrist to the mid-upper arm. The swelling is soft, there are no changes in colour or skin condition, and the shape is good.

Consider Julia's history and reflect upon the factors involved in the appearance of the swelling.

- What might have triggered Julia's swelling?
- What advice would you give her?

Julia is at risk of lymphoedema following her breast cancer treatment which included the removal of lymph nodes in her axilla. The initial swelling that she experienced following the surgery was of an acute nature, but it is likely that the radiotherapy to the chest wall has caused further acute inflammation in the area and could possibly compromise drainage of the lymphatic channels.

The increased exertion involved in unpacking boxes and moving furniture during the recent house move would have stimulated production of lymph fluid and, combined with the reduced lymph drainage routes from the arm, triggered swelling to appear in the tissues.

Julia should be advised that it is likely that she has early-onset lymphoedema caused by her breast cancer treatment and triggered by the recent exertive activity involved in moving house. The priority is to minimise further swelling and the following advice should be offered.

- Encourage lymph drainage by avoiding prolonged exertive activities such as carrying, pulling, pushing or lifting with the left arm. Carry out moderate activities for short periods only and stop if the arm begins to ache. Get help with the heavier tasks.
- Avoid infection by looking after the skin to ensure it is kept clean, healthy and intact at all times.
- The recording of simple surface measurements will give an indication of the degree of swelling that is present.
- A compression garment may be required to reduce the swelling that is present. It may not be required long term if Julia modifies her activities and the swelling settles quickly, but her risk of further swelling will always be present.

Case Scenario 2

Michael is a 48-year-old man who three weeks ago underwent a right groin dissection for recurrent melanoma in his right leg. Michael runs a public house and works long hours behind the bar. He was advised to take some time off work following his surgery, but one night a member of his bar staff had to go home because they were unwell. Michael went to help out and spent three hours on his feet behind the bar. The next day his right shoe did not fit and his leg was swollen. He rested his leg and the swelling slowly resolved. A week later he went to a rugby match with a group of friends. He had to stand during the train journey there and after the match they went for a drink and stood in the busy public house. The train was very full again on the way home, so he did not get a seat and by the time he got home his leg was aching. The next day he noticed it was swollen again and this time the swelling took longer to settle.

Consider Michael's history and reflect upon the factors involved in the appearance of his swelling.

- What might have triggered Michael's swelling?
- What advice would you give him?

The disruption to the lymphatic drainage routes in the groin caused by Michael's surgery places him at risk of developing lymphoedema. Michael should be advised that the history suggests that he has developed early-onset lymphoedema triggered by standing for long periods. This causes stasis of lymph fluid in the legs when the reduced action of the muscle pump is unable to encourage lymph drainage.

> The swelling appears to be of a transient nature because it settles over time. Michael should be offered the following advice.
>
> - Encourage lymph drainage by avoiding standing still for long periods. If standing is unavoidable, it should be for short periods of time only and some simple leg exercises at the time will stimulate the muscle pump and encourage lymph drainage.
> - If the leg begins to ache, it is better to rest in order to minimise any further problems.
> - Avoid infection by looking after the skin to ensure it is kept clean, healthy and intact at all times.
> - The recording of simple surface measurements will give an indication of the degree of any swelling that is present and provide information upon which future evaluation can be based.
> - A compression garment to minimise the further accumulation of lymph fluid may be required if the swelling recurs.

Conclusion

The recognition of early, uncomplicated lymphoedema is vital if progression to a more complex scenario is to be avoided. By identifying the risk factors, signs and clinical features of lymphoedema, the health-care professional can offer the patient early advice, information and support to enable them to manage any swelling.

References

Armer J., Radina E., Porock D. and Cuthbertson S. (2003) Predicting breast cancer-related lymphoedema using self-reported symptoms. *Nursing Research*, **52**(6): 370–9.

Board J. and Harlow W. (2002) Lymphoedema 2: classification, signs, symptoms and diagnosis. *British Journal of Nursing*, **11**(6): 389–95.

British Lymphology Society (2001) *Chronic Oedema: Population and Needs*. British Lymphology Society, Sevenoaks, Kent.

Clark B., Sitzia J. and Harlow W. (2005) Incidence and risk of arm oedema following treatment for breast cancer: a three year follow-up study. *Quarterly Journal of Medicine*, **98**(5): 343–8.

Foldi E. and Foldi M. (2003) Lymphostatic diseases. In: M. Foldi, E. Foldi and S. Kubik (eds) *Textbook of Lymphology for Physicians and Lymphoedema Therapists*. Urban and Fischer, Germany, pp. 232–319.

International Society of Lymphology (2000) The diagnosis and treatment of peripheral lymphoedema. Consensus document of the International Society of Lymphology. *Lymphology*, **36**(2): 84–91.

Katch V. and Weltman A. (1975) Predicatability of body segment volumes in living subjects. *Human Biology*, **47**(2): 203–18.

Keeley V. (2000) Clinical features of lymphoedema. In: R. Twycross, K. Jenns and J. Todd (eds) *Lymphoedema*. Radcliffe Medical Press, Oxford, pp. 44–67.

Kettle J., Rundle F. and Oddie T. (1958) Measurement of upper limb volumes: a clinical method. *Australian and New Zealand Journal of Surgery*, **27**(4): 263–70.

Kissin M.W., Querci della Rovere G., Easton D. and Westbury G. (1986) Risk of lymphoedema following the treatment of breast cancer. *British Journal of Surgery*, **73**: 580–4.

Mortimer P., Bates D., Brassington H., Stanton A., Strachan D. and Levick J. (1996) The prevalence of arm oedema following treatment of breast cancer. *Quarterly Journal of Medicine*, **89**: 377–80.

Piller N. (1999) Gaining an accurate assessment of the stages of lymphoedema subsequent to cancer: the role of objective and subjective information – when to make measurements and their optimal use. *European Journal of Lymphology*, **7**(25): 1–9.

Quade G. (2004) *Lymphoedema: Supportive Care Statement for Health Professionals*. Medical News: National Cancer Institute. Available at: www.cancer.gov (accessed 20/11/05).

Stanton A., Badger C. and Sitzia J. (2000) Non-invasive assessment of the lymphoedematous limb. *Lymphology*, **33**: 122–35.

Stanton A., Levick J. and Mortimer P. (1996) Current puzzles presented by postmastectomy oedema (breast cancer related lymphoedema). *Vascular Medicine*, **1**(3): 213–25.

5 A Framework for the Assessment of a Patient with Lymphoedema

Introduction

Lymphoedema is more than just swelling. It can influence quality of life and have a wider impact upon the patient's family and friends. The response to the development of lymphoedema is personal and unique; it may be a minor inconvenience for some but for others, lymphoedema can compromise lifestyle and make ordinary tasks difficult. A comprehensive and effective assessment of the patient should be a positive event, providing an opportunity to establish the impact of the swelling and enable priorities in its management to be highlighted at an early stage. This then forms the basis for planned, appropriate and timely intervention based upon the patient's needs.

The aim of this chapter is to highlight the importance of a comprehensive assessment of the patient with lymphoedema and how this can inform future care and management of the swelling.

Learning objectives

At the end of this chapter the reader will be able to:

- outline the principles of assessment
- discuss how the principles of assessment can be applied to an assessment of the patient with lymphoedema
- discuss the role of the health-care professional in assessing the patient with lymphoedema.

Principles of assessment

Rather than a single event, assessment is an ongoing activity during which the patient's needs are regularly reassessed, interventions are evaluated and the plan of care adjusted accordingly. Central to this process is the patient, who should play an active role in any assessment of their actual or potential needs, thus ensuring that the process remains patient focused and incorporates a holistic approach.

Assessment techniques vary according to the health-care setting. In the critical care setting, for example, assessment of the highly dependent patient will focus on vital signs while in the rehabilitation setting, the patient's quality of life becomes the focus. A structure for the assessment can be provided by nursing models but Murphy et al. (2000) warn that if the model chosen is inappropriate for the area of practice, the assessment information collected may be poorly utilised.

Webb (2004) outlines five stages in the assessment process which are based on the work of Alfaro-Lefevre (1999).

1. *Assessment.* To identify risk factors and actual patient needs.
2. *Problem identification.* To determine actual and potential problems combined with patient strengths and preferences.
3. *Planning.* To reduce risk factors, improve problems and utilise patient strengths.
4. *Implementation.* To determine the appropriateness of interventions and then implement and modify where required.
5. *Evaluation.* To assess progress, modify or stop the intervention.

An assessment of the patient should incorporate subjective and objective data. The inclusion of subjective data ensures patient participation and may include the patient's knowledge and awareness of their condition and current problem, a perception of previous interventions, personal feelings and available support networks (Webb 2004). It will also include the patient's perception of how the problem affects their quality of life. Objective data acquired from observation and measurement of the limbs provide a valuable tool for a later evaluation of the interventions implemented.

Principles of assessment applied to patients with lymphoedema

In lymphoedema management, elements of assessment are important for the following reasons.

● To distinguish between lymphoedema and other causes of oedema.

- To establish the extent and degree of the swelling and identify any complicating factors.
- To establish the effects that the swelling may have for the patient.
- To plan an individualised, realistic and appropriate treatment plan.

The assessment process outlined by Webb (2004) can be applied to an assessment of the patient with lymphoedema.

Assessment

A review of the patient's medical history will highlight any risk factors for the development of lymphoedema arising out of medical procedures or treatment involving lymph node areas. The type of treatment the patient has undergone should be noted, together with the commencement and completion dates and an indication of when the swelling developed. A history of the swelling to illustrate any changes and when these occur, together with consideration of the influence of any medications, should also be established. A probable cause for the swelling can then be determined, enabling the health-care professional to identify from the history obtained whether the patient is likely to have oedema or lymphoedema.

Problem identification

This part of the assessment can be considered within three areas in order to identify patient-focused problem areas.

1. *Physical assessment*. A physical assessment of the swollen area will help to identify the degree and extent of the swelling, the condition of the skin and whether the shape of the limb has been influenced by the swelling. It will also help to identify any complicating factors that may require further, more specialised advice and intervention. Aspects of a physical assessment are outlined in Table 5.1.
2. *Psychosocial assessment*. Establishing the influence of the swelling upon the patient's lifestyle, occupation and chosen social activities will help to identify problem areas that may require adjustment or adaptation in order to control the swelling. Aspects of a psychosocial assessment are outlined in Table 5.2.
3. *Psychological assessment*. This aspect of the assessment should include the impact of the lymphoedema in areas such as the patient's emotions, feelings about any changes in body image due to the swelling and any impact of the swelling upon relationships with family and friends. Aspects of a psychological assessment are outlined in Table 5.3.

Table 5.1   Aspects of a physical assessment of a patient with lymphoedema.

Aspect	How assessed	Rationale for the assessment
Assessment of the condition of the skin	History taking: • To identify any history of previous episodes of infection/skin conditions that may compromise skin integrity and place the patient at risk of future infections Examination of the limb: • To observe for any damage or breaks in the skin or signs of localised or systemic infection • To establish the colour, warmth and sensation of the limb	• To identify situations where skin integrity may be compromised, placing the patient at risk of infection. • To establish whether treatment for any infection is required. • To establish if there are venous or arterial considerations requiring further, more specialised assessment before any treatment plan is devised. • To establish whether the skin is fragile or broken and therefore unsuitable for the use of compression garments which may cause further damage. • To identify areas where patient education in skin care is required.
Assessment of the shape of the swollen limb	Examination of the limb: • To establish the distribution of the swelling and whether the normal shape of the limb has been influenced • To observe for any skin folds or creases occurring due to the swelling	• To establish potential problems with body image and the fitting of clothes. • To establish whether the use of compression garments is appropriate in the management of the patient's lymphoedema. • To become aware of all areas involved in the swelling so that treatment can be planned appropriately.
Assessment of the degree and extent of the swelling	Visual examination of the tissues surrounding the swollen area Palpation of the tissues to assess for any difference in the thickness	
Assessment of the size of the limb	Surface measurements of the limb. These may be simple or 4 cm volume measurements	• To form a baseline upon which to plan management of the swelling. • To provide measurements for future comparison and evaluation of the treatment plan.

Table 5.2   Aspects of a psychosocial assessment.

Aspect	How assessed	Rationale for the assessment
Assessment of limb function and discussion of the influence of the lymphoedema on the patient's limb movement, their day-to-day roles, hobbies, social activities and occupation	History taking: ● Adoption of a holistic approach, to listen to the patient's story in order to establish whether there are any specific areas of concern or difficulty Assessment of limb function: ● Observe for any difficulty with limb movement due to the size or weight of the limb ● Observe for a difficulty with limb function due to discomfort, pain or stiffness ● Observe for any difference in the sensation of the limb and surrounding tissues	● To identify situations where the swelling may already be influencing preferred activities so that appropriate advice can be given concerning these activities. ● To identify activities that may require modification, adaptation or avoidance in order to control the swelling. ● To identify whether referral to a member of the multiprofessional team is required in order to improve function or assist with activities of daily living. ● To identify areas where patient education in the use of their swollen limb is required to promote lymph drainage but minimise exertion and repetitive movements.

Planning

Following the identification of problem areas, appropriate strategies for the management of lymphoedema, applied to the patient's specific needs, can be discussed in order to formulate an individualised treatment plan. This will take into account the patient's medical history, knowledge of their condition, prognosis, motivation and their ability to take an active role in the management of their swelling. It may also include the participation of family members.

The planning should focus on objectives in order to address immediate priorities and also identify long- and short-term goals that are realistic, achievable and agreed by the patient.

Table 5.3   Aspects of a psychological assessment.

Aspect	How assessed	Rationale for the assessment
Assessment of the impact of the swelling upon the patient's feelings, emotions and relationships	History taking: ● Adopt a holistic approach, to establish whether there are any specific areas of concern or difficulty for the patient Listening and observation: ● Listen carefully to the patient's story and observe for signs of emotional distress, anger, depression or anxiety	● To establish whether the development of swelling has influenced relationships of a personal, sexual or social nature so that appropriate support and advice can be provided if necessary. ● To allow the patient time to express their concerns and explore ways of managing them. ● To establish whether the patient is receiving support from friends and family members so that ways of involving them can be explored if necessary. ● To establish whether referral to a member of the multiprofessional team is required in order to provide psychological support in dealing with the lymphoedema.

Implementation

As lymphoedema is a chronic condition, implementation of the care discussed will rely on the patient becoming an active participant in the management of their swelling. Factors involved in the success of this aspect of the assessment include the patient's understanding of what they have agreed to do and why it is included in their care. Positive motivational factors and support from friends and family are also crucial factors involved in the successful implementation of care.

Evaluation

Once lymphoedema has developed, its management is life-long in order to control the swelling. Regular, ongoing evaluation of management strategies is therefore an essential aspect of care and helps to ensure that treatment remains appropriate and patient focused. It also ensures that the patient feels supported in managing their swelling and enables early identification of any subsequent complicating factors that may develop.

The role of the health-care professional in assessment

The development of lymphoedema is perceived in a unique manner by each patient. Response to the condition may be influenced by past experience – perhaps that of colleagues, family members or friends with oedema. It is also influenced by knowledge and understanding of the condition gained from a variety of sources. A mixture of feelings, thoughts and beliefs is therefore brought to the assessment to be utilised in the development of a holistic treatment plan, facilitated by a skilled health-care professional.

The health-care professional also holds perceptions, beliefs and levels of knowledge concerning lymphoedema, acquired through their own experience, both professional and personal. These perceptions influence their interpretation of the patient's needs and, when considered within the concepts of philosophy, knowledge and theory, can provide a background to the assessment process (Woods 2002).

Philosophy

A philosophical approach to the assessment of a patient with lymphoedema involves recognition of the patient as an individual (Woods 2002). During interaction with the patient, the health-care professional gathers information but moves away from the scientific approach adopted during the assessment, such as the use of limb measurements, to develop a more personal understanding of what it is like for the patient to have lymphoedema and the impact it may be having. By adopting an individual, holistic approach, the health-care professional can work in partnership with the patient and begin to empower them to take appropriate action to manage their swelling and make adjustments to ensure its long-term control. This may involve education and support to make personal changes which may be necessary to minimise the risk of complications developing, or acting on a more collective level through self-help support groups to gain additional advice and support from other lymphoedema sufferers.

Knowledge

During the assessment, the health-care professional will blend several forms of knowledge acquired from different sources to achieve the aim of a holistic assessment with an individualised treatment plan. Carper (1978) outlines different types of knowledge which can be observed in an assessment of a patient with lymphoedema.

Skilled knowledge

Professional experience and training will lead to skilled knowledge, enabling the health-care professional to recognise lymphoedema and understand its development. Information obtained from the patient's medical history coupled with a physical examination of the affected area are crucial components of this part of the assessment.

Aesthetic knowledge

Skilled knowledge is then applied creatively according to the individual situation. Combining ethical and analytical considerations with empathy and evidence-based practice, the health-care professional will channel skilled knowledge into an interpretation of the patient's needs and the development of an appropriate treatment plan.

Intuitive knowledge

Intuition is viewed by Benner (1984) as a feature of expert practice. Difficult to define and primarily based on perceptions of a situation, it can be considered an important element of the assessment of a patient with lymphoedema. The health-care professional interprets verbal and non-verbal cues to gain an understanding of the meaning of lymphoedema for the patient and develop a perception of the outcome of any intervention.

Lay knowledge

A considerable amount of information on health-care topics is now readily available to patients via a wide variety of sources and can provide valuable depth to a subject area to enhance understanding. However, information acquired in this manner can also be inappropriate for a patient's particular circumstances or conflict with information acquired elsewhere. During the assessment of a patient with lymphoedema, the health-care professional needs to establish the patient's current understanding of their condition to ensure that it is accurate and can be applied to an appropriate treatment plan.

Theory

The theory or evidence base for aspects of lymphoedema management is related to the physiology of the lymphatic system and the health-care professional requires knowledge concerning this to support treatment decisions made with the patient at the time of assessment. For example, the patient with lymphoedema is at increased risk of infection in the swollen area due to stasis of lymph fluid. The health-care professional will provide advice regarding skin care in order to minimise the risk of infection developing in the swollen area. The health-care professional will also be required to adapt their knowledge of lymphoedema management to the patient's particular circumstances and recognise when aspects of management are not required or are inappropriate. Locally developed clinical guidelines can also be used to support practice.

The following case scenarios highlight the importance of completing a thorough assessment of patients with lymphoedema in order to create an appropriate individualised treatment plan.

Case Scenario 1

When he was 11 years old, on holiday with his family in the Mediterranean, a mosquito bit Joel on his right ankle. The ankle initially became red and puffy but the discolouration settled after a few days, leaving a slight swelling in his right ankle. Joel paid very little attention to this as his leg was covered most of the time and the swelling was minimal.

Three years later, Joel was picked to represent his county at rugby and sustained a large gash on his right shin in the tournament, requiring stitching in the local casualty department. This took a while to heal but symptoms of redness, soreness and fever accompanied the trauma to his leg. As the injury healed, Joel noticed that the mild swelling that had previously just been in his ankle had become more extensive, with swelling in the foot, ankle and shin. Joel also noticed that the swelling subsided slightly when he was on holiday from school and less active, but his leg was always at its worst at the beginning of the week. He continued to play rugby every weekend and was a valued team player.

When he reached 20 years of age, Joel developed a further infection in his leg after he had a tattoo on his right thigh. This time the infection was worse than before and he was admitted to hospital for intravenous antibiotics. On admission, his leg was hot, red, swollen and tender and he was unwell with a high temperature. He was unable to get his slipper on his right foot and his pyjama trousers were tight along the length of his right leg. Joel had to cancel a rugby tour due to this admission to hospital and was not pleased about letting the team down. He asks you for more information about his swelling and the treatments that are available.

Reflect on what you know of Joel and identify key points relating to his swelling.

- What do you think might be the cause of Joel's swelling?
- What do you think are Joel's immediate physical needs?
- What impact do you think a diagnosis of lymphoedema will have upon Joel?
- What advice will Joel and his family require?

Joel's history suggests that his swelling is of non-cancer origin. He does not have a history of cancer or its treatment and is a young, fit and active man. In the absence of any other medical symptoms, further medical investigations should be carried out to establish if the swelling is due to primary lymphoedema.

Joel's immediate physical needs during this admission are to abolish the infection. As swelling is already present in the leg, and therefore stasis of lymphatic fluid has developed, a prolonged course of antibiotics will be required to ensure that the infection is effectively eradicated. Joel also needs advice concerning the care of his leg to ensure that the risk of future episodes of infection is minimised. This will include skin care to promote skin integrity and advice concerning management of the swelling.

Joel is a young man who is unlikely to welcome specific health-care needs into his daily life. He is a team player for whom the game of rugby is important and will have concerns regarding the continuity of his sport and his place within the rugby team. A change to important aspects of his life will feel threatening and could lead to social isolation.

Joel will need careful education and support to enable him to explore how he can accommodate his hobbies and activities into daily life with lymphoedema while minimising the risk of further infective episodes and potentially more problematic swelling.

Case Scenario 2

Beatrice is 78 years of age and has recurrent breast cancer with a large fungating tumour in her left axilla. She is receiving palliative chemotherapy which she knows will not cure her cancer, but she hopes that it will take away some of her discomfort.

Beatrice has swelling in her left hand, arm and chest wall. Her arm feels heavy and lifeless and it aches all the time like a bad toothache. The fungating tumour in her axilla requires daily dressings and Beatrice finds this procedure very distressing because it is painful to hold her arm in position as the dressings are being done. She cannot tolerate any pressure on her arm, even from clothes, and the swelling makes it difficult for her to do anything. Her husband is supportive and able to help at home but Beatrice is frustrated that she is unable to do anything because she is uncomfortable and limited by her swollen arm.

Reflect on what you know of Beatrice and identify key points relating to her swelling.

- What do you think might be the cause of Beatrice's swelling?
- What do you think are Beatrice's immediate physical needs?
- What impact do you think the lymphoedema is having upon Beatrice and her husband?

Beatrice's history indicates that the large fungating tumour in her axilla has caused an obstruction in the regional lymph nodes and a subsequent reduction in the lymphatic system transport capacity. Lymphoedema has developed in the hand, arm and chest wall area because of this obstruction.

Beatrice's immediate physical need will be appropriate pain relief to ensure that the daily dressings are completed without pain or discomfort. Adequate pain relief will also enable her to move her arm more and facilitate an improvement in her quality of life. The stasis of lymph fluid in the arm places her at risk of infection, so the promotion of skin integrity through an appropriate skin care regime will also be essential. Once the pain is controlled, gentle arm movements will encourage joint mobility and promote lymph movement.

Beatrice has advanced disease with a fungating tumour and lymphoedema. The visible swelling and difficulty with the use of her arm are likely to cause considerable distress as Beatrice becomes increasingly dependent upon her husband and unable to fulfil her previous roles in their relationship. The visible swelling and daily dressings to the tumour will remind her of her cancer and her inevitable mortality from its effects. Beatrice and her husband will require support and skilled care to ensure that priorities in the management of their needs are sensitively addressed by all members of the multiprofessional team.

Conclusion

The impact of the development of lymphoedema for the individual, their family and friends can be considerable. At the time of assessment, the health-care professional is challenged to listen to the patient's story and develop an understanding of their needs so that a clear pathway of management can be identified.

Although models of patient assessment vary according to circumstances, the needs of the patient with lymphoedema can best be considered within a holistic framework in which actual and potential needs are identified and the patient is encouraged to play an active role. Lymphoedema is a chronic condition with life-long implications. This chapter has considered a model of patient assessment utilising clinical skills and professional knowledge, coupled with recognition of the patient's unique contribution to control of the swelling and its future management.

References

Alfaro-Lefevre R. (1999) *Critical Thinking in Nursing: a practical approach*, 2nd edn. W.B. Saunders, Philadelphia.

Benner P. (1984) *From Novice to Expert: excellence and power in clinical nursing practice*. Addison-Wesley, Menlo Park.

Carper B. (1978) Fundamental ways of knowing in nursing. *Advanced Nursing Science*, **1**(1): 13–23.

Murphy K., Cooney A., Casey D., Connor M., O'Connor J. and Dineen B. (2000) The Roper, Logan and Tierney (1996) model: perceptions and operationalization of the model in psychiatric nursing within a Health Board in Ireland. *Journal of Advanced Nursing*, **31**(6): 1333–41.

Webb C. (2004) Communication and assessment. In: L. Dougherty and S. Lister (eds) *The Royal Marsden Manual of Clinical Nursing Procedures*, 6th edn. Blackwell Publishing, Oxford, pp. 27–37.

Woods M. (2002) Using philosophy, knowledge and theory to assess a patient with lymphoedema. *International Journal of Palliative Nursing*, **8**(4): 176–81.

6 Care of the Skin

Introduction

The skin is the largest and most visible organ in the body because it covers the exterior surface of the body (Kumar & Clark 2005). Accounting for approximately 15% of body weight, the skin is a complex structure composed of different layers which cover and protect underlying muscles and organs.

The skin is the body's first line of defence against many types of infections and it acts as a cushion against injury to the body. Maintaining its integrity is essential in the prevention of infection and promotion of health. Regeneration of the skin is a normal physiological process repeated approximately every 28 days. This process requires daily skin hygiene in order to keep the skin clean and prevent a build-up of dead skin, sweat and dirt on the skin surface. The functions of the skin become disturbed if it is allowed to become dirty, making it more prone to infections.

The lymphatic vessels have an important function in the immune surveillance of the body, clearing substances which penetrate the skin and controlling the microcirculation of the skin. When lymph drainage is reduced, normal function becomes disturbed. There is an increased risk of infection if the body's defences through the skin are breached and fluid, proteins and other macromolecules stagnate in the tissues due to the decreased lymph flow.

This aim of this chapter is to consider the normal physiology and function of the skin and how this is influenced when lymph drainage is reduced, so that the health-care professional can gain an understanding of the importance of a good skin care regime and be able to advise patients with lymphoedema concerning the care of their skin.

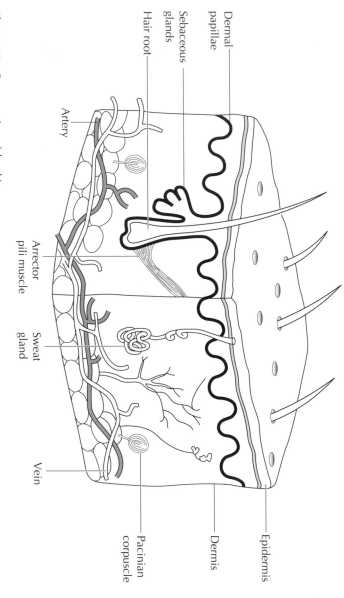

Dermal
papillae

Sebaceous
glands

Hair root

Artery

Arrector
pili muscle

Sweat
gland

Vein

Pacinian
corpuscle

Dermis

Epidermis

Figure 6.1 Cross-section of the skin.

Learning objectives

At the end of this chapter, the reader will be able to:

- describe the normal appearance, physiology and function of the skin
- discuss the effect of lymphoedema upon the skin
- outline and discuss the rationale for the care of the skin in a limb with, or at risk of, lymphoedema
- demonstrate an understanding of common and complex skin conditions that can occur in lymphoedema
- discuss the signs, symptoms and management of acute inflammatory episodes and their implications for the patient with lymphoedema.

Physiology and function of the skin

The skin is composed of three layers, as illustrated in Figure 6.1, and has several functions which are summarised in Table 6.1.

The epidermis

This is the outer layer of the skin which is especially thick on the soles of the feet and the palm of the hands. It is made up of five layers of cells, which do not contain blood vessels but are supplied with lymph fluid in the deeper layers (Marieb 2005). The outer layer is the protective layer of the skin in which cells are continually rubbed off by friction and replaced by new cells produced in the innermost layer, which then migrate towards the outer layers of the epidermis as they mature. The skin is protected against water loss and the absorption of harmful chemicals and pathogens by the outer layer of the epidermis.

The dermis

The dermis lies below the epidermis and is a tough, elastic layer that consists of loose connective tissue and contains a number of structures. These include blood vessels, lymphatic capillaries, sweat glands, hair follicles and sensory nerve endings. The dermis comprises two layers: the upper layer is made up of fine collagen and elastin fibres which are folded into ridges. These are especially noticeable on the palms of the hand and the soles of the feet. The lower layer contains more dense connective tissue and many thick collagen fibres.

Table 6.1 Functions of the skin.

Function	Why this is necessary	How this is achieved
Protection	• To protect the internal structures from physical injury • To protect the body from dehydration and excessive water absorption • To protect the body from the penetration of substances through the skin surface and invasion by micro-organisms • To protect the body from damage by ultraviolet rays from the sun	• The subcutaneous layer contains fat cells which act as padding for the body. • The epidermis retains water in the body whilst natural oils on the skin maintain water resistance. • The waxy nature of the surface of the skin and the natural surface secretions provide a protective function from the invasion of microorganisms. • Synthesis of vitamin D and vitamin B provides pigmentation to the skin to protect it from the effects of ultraviolet rays in sunlight.
Sensory perception	• To facilitate communication with our external environment • To alert the body to potential danger or injury	• Sensory receptors and nerves in the dermis layer enable us to experience sociosexual and emotional sensations. • Sensory receptors alert the body to the stimuli of pain and pressure.
Temperature regulation	• Control of body temperature is essential for the maintenance of health	• Excess heat is lost through the evaporation of sweat and the radiation of heat away from the body. • The body is insulated with subcutaneous fat to conserve heat and covered with hairs which provide an insulating layer on the skin when the body is cold. • Blood vessels in the skin dilate and constrict to control heat loss.

The subcutaneous layer

The subcutaneous layer lies below the dermis and consists of connective tissue and fat cells, interlaced with blood vessels. It provides a supportive structure for the outer layers of the skin and maintains regulation of the body temperature (Allen et al. 2004).

Healthy skin

To ensure that the skin is kept healthy, a balanced state of physiological conditions must exist. Although the skin can adapt to changes in the environment and overall health, the delicate balance between its physiological functions is dependent upon the maintenance of skin integrity and cleanliness.

Healthy skin has:

- a clear appearance
- an even colour
- a soft, supple texture when touched
- warmth, without surface moisture or greasiness
- a high degree of elasticity.

Failure to care for the skin can lead to damage and premature ageing. With increasing age, skin naturally becomes thinner as ridges in the dermis begin to flatten and the growth of epidermal and dermal cells slows down. Skin tears are possible as the skin becomes drier and as elasticity decreases and blood flow reduces, the body's first line of defence can become weakened. There is an increased risk of infection entering the body through a more permeable epidermis and tissue breakdown can occur through damage or injury (Allen et al. 2004).

Substances which penetrate the skin, such as topical drugs and medication, creams and cosmetics, are cleared away by the superficial initial lymphatics (Linnett 2000). Unwanted substances, such as microorganisms, can also penetrate the skin and are carried away by the superficial lymphatics to the lymph nodes which act as disposal centres to ensure the safety of the body.

The effect of lymphoedema upon the skin

Any disruption in the transport capacity of the regional lymph nodes will have an effect upon the lymph channels draining into the area and initiate a build-up of lymph fluid in the tissues. As fluid stasis develops, substances which penetrate the surface of the skin accumulate with lymph fluid in the tissues and trigger an inflammatory response. This leads to a reduction in

Table 6.2   Skin changes in lymphoedema.

Skin changes	Effect
The skin begins to thicken as lymphatic fluid slows down within the tissues.	It becomes difficult to pick up or pinch a fold of skin at the base of the fingers or toes. Stemmer's sign is positive.
Dilated lymph vessels in the superficial dermis bulge on the skin surface.	Called lymphangiomas, the dilated lymph vessels give the appearance of blisters and can leak lymph fluid if they become damaged, making the area prone to infection.
Skin thickening progresses as fibrin and collagen stagnate within the subcutaneous tissues.	Indentation of the tissues when pressed (pitting) becomes more difficult.
Fibrotic changes in the subcutaneous tissues progress.	The skin develops a brawny appearance and the tissues develop a solid consistency.
A horny scale builds up on the surface of the skin, termed hyperkeratosis.	Skin creases develop where hyperkeratosis is present with an increase in microorganisms in the warm moist environment they create. The risk of fungal and bacterial infections developing is high.
Dilated skin lymphatics surrounded by rigid fibrous tissue protrude from the skin as papules or nodules, termed papillomatosis.	A cobblestone appearance develops on the skin surface.
Connective tissue growth increases due to stagnation of plasma proteins and the stratum corneum in the epithelium continues to thicken.	The skin loses its elasticity and the shape of the limb becomes altered.

macrophage activity and an overgrowth of interstitial connective tissue (Williams & Venables 1996). The skin begins to lose its natural elasticity and with time, the progressive effect upon the skin becomes visible, although the rate of change varies considerably between patients (Keeley 2000). Table 6.2 outlines the changes that occur in the skin when lymphoedema is present and describes the effects of lymph stasis.

Microorganisms can breach the body's defences when the local immune response has been compromised following cancer treatment involving local lymph node areas and the ability of the lymphatic channels to clear away substances becomes reduced. If a bacterial infection enters through a break in the skin, the inflammatory response of the body will increase lymph load and a worsening of the swelling is accompanied by pain and discomfort in the limb, with systemic symptoms which can be severe in nature. Acute inflammatory episodes are discussed later in this chapter.

Caring for the skin

A good skin care regime is a vital part of the management of lymphoedema aimed at achieving healthy, clean, well-moisturised and intact skin. Health-care professionals should be able to assess the skin and identify any problems so that patients can be advised regarding management of their skin. All patients with, or at risk of, lymphoedema should be encouraged to adopt a daily skin care regime to promote skin integrity and reduce the risk of infection.

Skin assessment and observation

By examining the skin daily, the patient will develop an awareness of any changes in the condition of the skin and notice any cuts, breaks or accidental trauma which may occur so that these can be treated promptly with an antiseptic cream to minimise the risk of infection.

Two skin assessment tools, which are not currently validated, have been proposed for use within lymphoedema management to assist health-care professionals in their assessment of a patient's skin. Linnett (2000) proposed a simple grading system to assist in measuring the outcome of skin care according to the physical condition of the skin established on visual examination. An earlier scoring system was proposed by Badger & Jeffs (1995) to consider the condition of the skin and subcutaneous tissues in relation to the site of the swelling, the shape and size of the limb. In this assessment tool a score is calculated from the assessment in order to evaluate the effect of lymphoedema management.

While grading or scoring tools can be useful in assessing the condition of the skin and evaluating the outcome of skin care, subjective assessment by the patient and health-care professional remains vital and should include the wider impact of the skin's condition upon the patient. A poor skin condition with associated problems can cause discomfort and influence quality of life. The health-care professional should work with the patient to improve the condition of the skin where necessary, by providing appropriate information to promote and maintain skin integrity and considering the patient's individual needs.

The treatment of any underlying skin conditions should be a priority in lymphoedema management as these may influence the outcome of care (Mortimer 1995). The disease status of patients with a cancer diagnosis should always be established in order to assess whether skin problems may be related to disease progression (Maclaren 2001).

Palpation of the skin should always accompany a visual examination and will reveal whether the skin is hot – a symptom which may imply infection or chronic inflammation (Linnett 2000). Palpation will also indicate the condition of the subcutaneous tissues.

Skin cleansing

Gentle, daily cleansing of the skin should aim to remove pathogenic organisms, dust and dirt but not be so vigorous that natural oils which protect the skin are also removed (Penzer 2003). A mild, unperfumed soap or soap substitute such as aqueous cream is preferred and abrasive soaps should be avoided.

Care should be taken when drying the skin. Rubbing will disturb the skin barrier function and should be replaced by patting of the skin during drying, taking care to dry the skin thoroughly. Particular attention should be paid to skin creases or folds and the spaces between the digits or toes where residual moisture in a warm environment can lead to fungal infections.

Skin moisturising

The daily moisturising of skin in an area where lymphoedema is present or possible will encourage moisture to be retained by the skin and skin integrity to be promoted. Any dryness, flaking or cracking of the skin indicates that the skin is no longer intact and the increased colonisation of potentially harmful bacteria in dry skin may compound the reduced immunity of the limb and increase the risk of infection developing. Moisturising of the skin is therefore important for all patients with, or at risk of, lymphoedema, to prevent dryness occurring.

An emollient agent is recommended for use in moisturising the limb (Linnett 2000, Maclaren 2001, Williams & Venables 1996). Emollients provide a surface lipid film to the epidermis which prevents water loss from the skin and reduces the risk of dryness (Williams & Venables 1996).

Emollients can be divided into three categories.

- *Bath oils*. These help to restore the integrity of the skin and prevent it from drying out.
- *Soap substitutes*. These can be mixed with water to provide a liquid soap with an oil and water content and should be used in conjunction with an emollient cream to rehydrate the skin if it is very dry.
- *Moisturisers*. These may be in the form of lotions, creams or ointments.

The choice of emollient depends upon the condition of the skin and Linnett (2000) proposed a three-step ladder, summarised here, to assist in the choice of suitable emollient.

- Well-hydrated skin requires a bland moisturising emollient in the form of a lotion or cream which is easily applied and absorbed.
- Dry, flaky skin requires an emollient ointment which is greasy and forms an impermeable layer over the skin.
- Scaly/hyperkeratotic skin requires a soap substitute and moisturising ointment to soften the areas involved so that they can be removed.

Moisturising with an appropriate emollient is an important, life-long aspect of care that all patients with, or at risk of, lymphoedema should incorporate into their daily routine. Patient preference will need to be considered in the choice of agent and will encourage compliance, but a clear rationale for the type of emollient recommended will need to be discussed.

Emollients should usually be applied once a day but when the skin is scaly and hyperkeratotic, a twice-daily application is preferred. Applying the emollient liberally to the skin at night will ensure that the skin benefits from its application before any compression garments are fitted the next morning. The moisturiser should be applied to the whole of the limb and adjacent part of the trunk, with the last movement carried out downwards in the direction of the hair growth. This ensures that the moisturiser does not accumulate in the hair follicles which can lead to a condition called folliculitis in which there is inflammation of the hair follicles and sometimes infection.

Common skin problems

A number of skin problems can occur when lymphoedema has developed. Table 6.3 presents a summary of the features and management of those discussed here.

Dry skin

Dryness of the skin can develop as a result of irritants in the environment or as the natural ageing process reduces the elasticity and pliability of the skin. In lymphoedema, the skin becomes stretched and can then become dry, rough and scaly with visible flaking.

Dry skin feels tight, rough and itchy. It tightens after washing and fine lines can be observed on the surface. At its worst, dry skin may develop cracks and be painful. Bacteria colonise on dry flaky skin and infection may develop in the area if cracks in the skin occur through dryness.

Table 6.3   Skin conditions and their management.

Skin condition	Appearance	Management
Dry skin	Tight, rough, flaky skin	Daily application of an emollient ointment
Folliculitis	Small inflamed pimples or pustules on the skin near a hair follicle	Skin cleansing followed by the application of emollient with the last movement downward towards the direction of hair growth
Fungal infections (tinea pedis)	Itchy, flaky or macerated skin in the web spaces of the toes	Skin cleansing and use of an antifungal cream
Hyperkeratosis	Thickened warty, scaly skin with a brown/grey appearance	Daily or twice-daily application of an emollient ointment. Salicylic acid to small areas with care
Papillomatosis	Hardened papules or nodules on the surface of the skin giving a cobblestone appearance	Regular application of emollients. Compression bandages can be useful
Lymphangioma	Small, fragile lymph blisters on the surface of the skin	Scrupulous skin cleansing and avoidance of trauma. May require surgical cautery if repeated leakage leads to infection
Acute inflammatory episodes	Sudden onset of fever, shivering, headaches and nausea associated with localised symptoms of pain, rash, inflammation and increased swelling in the swollen limb	Antibiotics for a minimum of 14 days and rest until the acute phase has passed

Treatment involves the use of an emollient ointment to form an impermeable layer over the skin and prevent loss of moisture, and the skin should be protected from the drying elements of the sun, wind and cold.

Folliculitis

Folliculitis is inflammation of one or more hair follicles (Linnett 2000) identified by the appearance of small inflamed pimples or pustules appearing on the skin near a hair follicle. It can occur when the hair follicles become blocked with greasy moisturisers and if allowed to progress, will lead to an

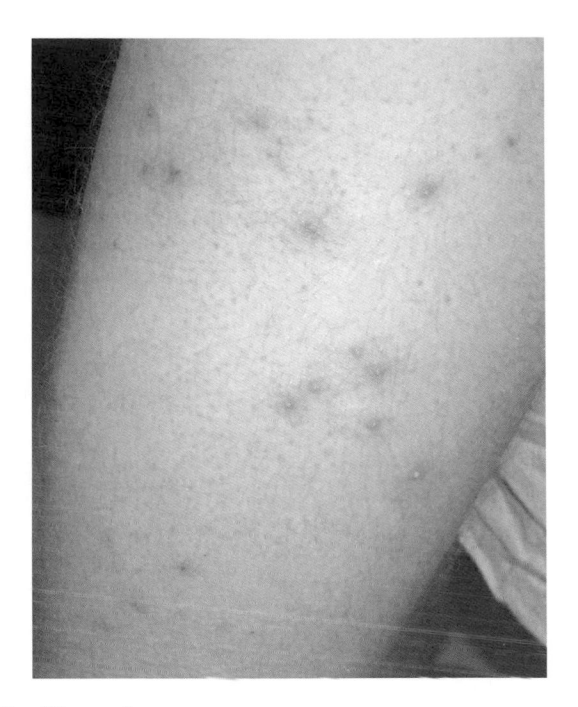

Figure 6.2   Folliculitis on a leg.

infection of the blocked follicles. Figure 6.2 highlights folliculitis which developed on a leg.

Treatment involves careful cleansing of the skin followed by the application of an appropriate amount of emollient applied in a thorough manner. Once the emollient has been rubbed into the skin, the last movement should be downward in the direction of hair growth (Linnett 2000). This will ensure that emollient residue is not left trapped in the hair follicle.

Fungal infections

Fungal infections can develop where swollen skin is dry and flaky or moist and macerated (Board & Harlow 2002). The web spaces between swollen toes enclosed within socks and footwear provide an ideal environment for a fungal infection known as tinea pedis to develop and secondary infections from bacteria entering into the subcutaneous tissues through broken skin can further complicate the condition. The condition often causes intense itching in the area infected and the skin may appear flaky and macerated. Figure 6.3 illustrates a fungal infection between the toes.

Treatment involves meticulous skin hygiene with careful drying between the toes and the wearing of clean, cotton socks. A topical antifungal powder

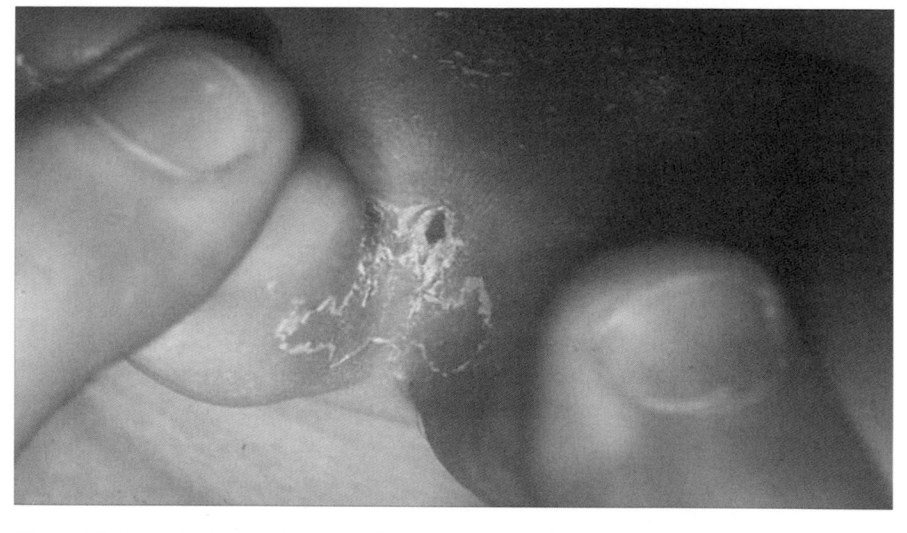

Figure 6.3 Fungal infection between the toes.

or cream should be applied every day until the infection has cleared and diligence is required to ensure the condition does not recur.

Complex skin problems

In more advanced lymphoedema, characteristic skin changes can often be observed.

Hyperkeratosis

The continued stasis of lymph fluid in the tissues triggers an inflammatory response and as fibrin and collagen are deposited, an increased thickening of the stratum corneum within the epidermis occurs. The skin becomes thick, hard and woody in texture and appears warty with brown/grey scale-like changes.

The condition is more commonly seen in patients with lower limb lymphoedema because of the added influence of gravity and the skin changes may be particularly evident on the feet. Figure 6.4 illustrates hyperkeratosis occurring on the leg.

Regular, daily or twice-daily application of an emollient ointment will soften and lift the hardened skin. A keratotic agent such as Diprosalic ointment (salicylic acid) can be useful in small areas to break down particularly hardened skin but must be used with care due to the risk of skin irritation (Maclaren 2001). Once the condition of the skin has improved, a bland moisturising emollient can be used to maintain hydration of the skin.

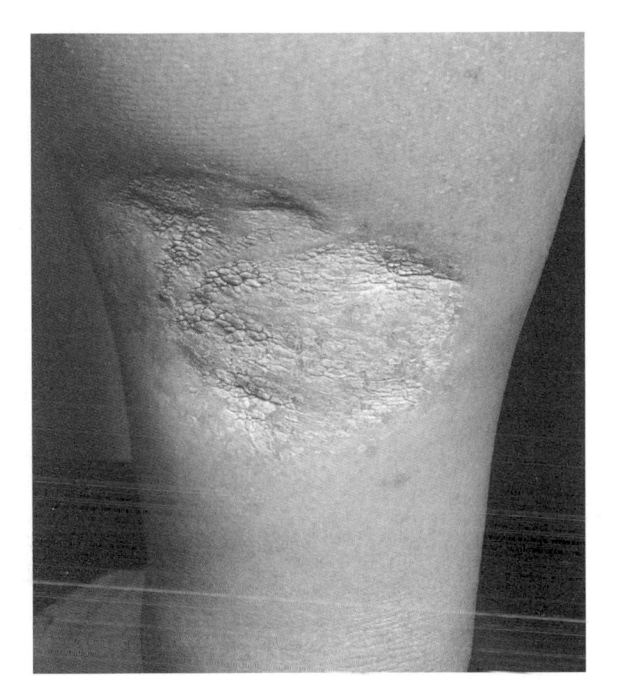

Figure 6.4   Hyperkeratosis on a leg where a melanoma has previously been excised.

Papillomatosis

Where hyperkeratosis exists, there may also be the development of raised projections on the skin which contain dilated lymphatics. These give a cobblestone appearance to the skin, which takes on a rough, uneven texture, and are caused by cutaneous fibrosis. Figure 6.5 illustrates papillomatosis occurring in the leg.

Management involves scrupulous skin cleansing and the prevention of skin trauma, particularly whilst applying or removing compression garments. The skin should be moisturised with an emollient ointment and the condition can be greatly improved with the use of compression bandages which apply a firm pressure to the skin.

Lymphangioma

Superficial, dilated lymph vessels can herniate through the epithelial layer of the skin to appear as small lymph blisters. These may be singular or in clusters and are filled with clear lymph fluid. The blisters are very fragile and if damaged they will leak, posing a risk of infection. Figure 6.6 illustrates the appearance of lymphangioma.

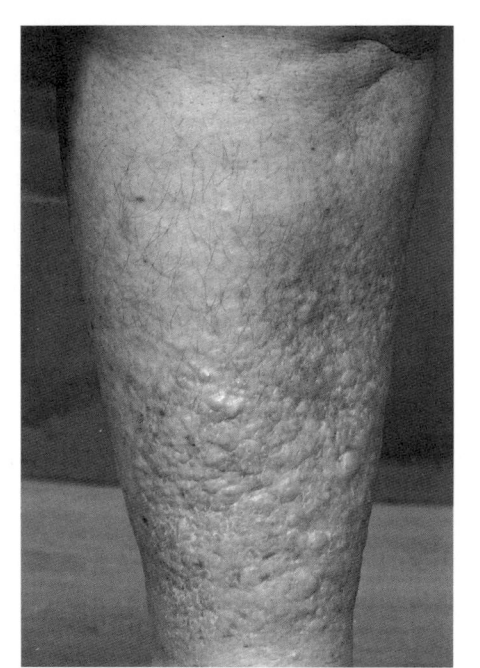

Figure 6.5 Papillomatosis in a leg.

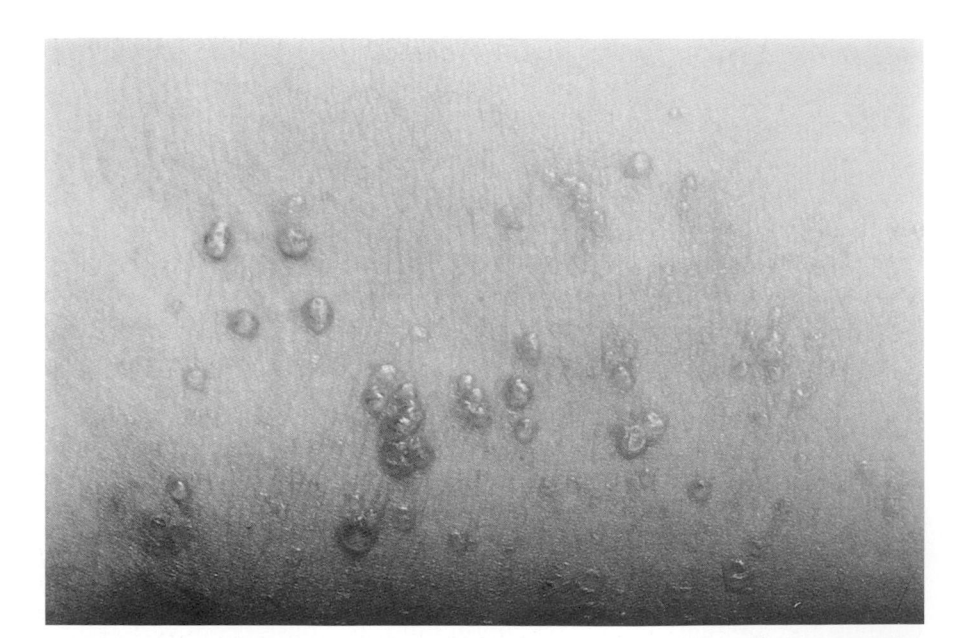

Figure 6.6 Lymphangioma.

The management of areas where lymphangiomas are present involves scrupulous skin cleansing and moisturising to promote skin integrity. Compression can be helpful in encouraging the dilated lymphatics to flatten, but surgical cauterisation may be required if the problem persists and causes recurrent infection.

Acute inflammatory episodes

A frequently reported feature of lymphoedema is the development of acute episodes of apparent infection which follow a characteristic clinical picture. The term used to describe these episodes varies considerably in the literature and can lead to some confusion. Authors refer to:

- acute inflammatory episodes (Mortimer 2000)
- cellulitis (LSN 2006, Woo et al. 2000)
- erysipelas (Foldi & Foldi 2003, Masmoudi et al. 2005).

Description

An acute inflammatory episode is characterised by a sudden onset of systemic symptoms such as fever, shivering, headaches and nausea which are associated with localised symptoms of pain, rash, inflammation and increased swelling in the swollen limb. The patient may recall a recent trauma or skin puncture to the affected limb but in many cases a cause for the development of the episode cannot be established.

The presenting symptoms vary between patients. While some patients experience relatively mild symptoms, others quickly become very ill and require hospitalisation. Recovery can take several days or weeks and if the condition does not fully resolve, recurrent episodes can occur. Figure 6.7 highlights how a severe acute inflammatory episode may present in a leg.

Cause

The cause of acute inflammatory episodes is widely considered to be bacterial in origin (Board & Harlow 2002, Foldi & Foldi, 2003, Maclaren 2001, Masmoudi et al. 2005, Woo et al. 2000), resulting from the infective organism group B streptococcus (Masmoudi et al. 2005). Due to a reduction in lymph drainage, it is thought that the bacteria breach the body's defences to thrive in the lack of local immunity and rapidly spread throughout the tissues. In many cases, however, a causative organism cannot be isolated

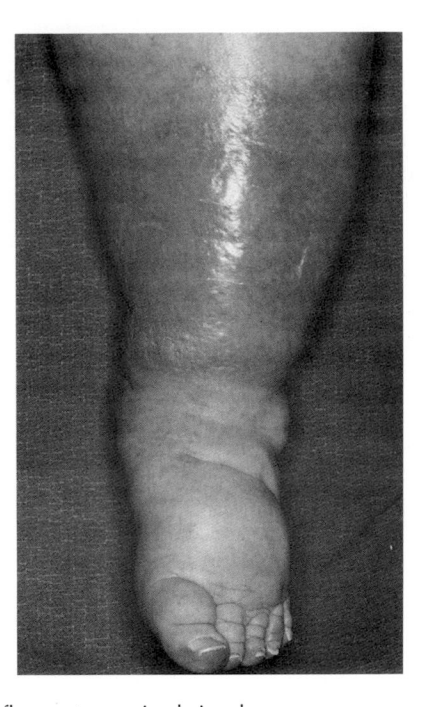

Figure 6.7   An acute inflammatory episode in a leg.

(Mortimer 2000) and some patients report an association with circumstances unrelated to a skin puncture where skin integrity has been preserved. It is therefore clear that the cause of acute inflammatory episodes is more complex than a bacterial infection.

Incidence

Any breach of skin integrity, including the presence of dry, flaky skin on a swollen limb, is considered a risk for the development of infection. Studies have shown that acute inflammatory episodes are more likely to occur the longer lymphoedema has been present and when it is more chronic in nature (Mortimer 2000). Many patients who experience an acute inflammatory episode suffer recurrent episodes and begin a vicious cycle where their swelling worsens with each recurrent attack.

Management

All patients with, or at risk of, lymphoedema should be advised about the possibility of acute inflammatory episodes. Good skin hygiene and moisturising will reduce the risk of skin damage and the possibility of bacterial infiltration of the tissues, while the avoidance of exertive, strenuous activities will reduce the risk of an inflammatory response to injury which can then lead to an acute inflammatory episode.

Patients should be alert to the signs and symptoms of an attack so that medical advice can be sought and treatment started as early as possible. Antibiotics are given orally unless the patient has rapidly become unwell, in which case intravenous antibiotics may be required.

A consensus on the medical management of acute inflammatory episodes was recently reached between health-care professionals and medical practitioners in the UK which states the appropriate antibiotics to be used, dosage and course duration to be followed if an attack occurs (BLS and LSN 2005). If patients suffer recurrent attacks, long-term prophylactic antibiotic use is recommended and has been shown to be effective in minimising further attacks (Mortimer 2000).

Implications

Acute inflammatory episodes, particularly when they are recurrent, can have a negative impact upon the patient's swelling and their quality of life. With each attack, the swelling in the limb can progress and although the acute nature of the swelling will settle once the attack is treated, residual swelling may remain, with the result that the limb size is greater than before the attack.

During an attack the patient will be ill, necessitating a change in routine activities which may have work or lifestyle implications. Rest is essential until the acute phase has passed and it may take as long as a few months for the attack to completely resolve.

The following case scenarios illustrate the importance of good skin care for patients who have lymphoedema.

Case Scenario 1

Rob is a 40-year-old man who is a carpenter by trade but also works with his friend in his painting and decorating business. Two years ago Rob underwent removal of the lymph glands in his right axilla following a diagnosis of non-Hodgkin's lymphoma. Since then Rob has had some mild lymphoedema in his arm. He reluctantly wears a compression sleeve when he is working, but does not want to use greasy creams on his skin. On holiday recently, he got sunburnt and his skin is now dry and flaky.

Reflect on what you know of Rob's history.

- Why has Rob got dry, flaky skin?
- What skin care advice should he be given?

Because Rob has lymphoedema in his right arm, the skin is susceptible to the effects of lymph stasis in the tissues and is prone to dryness. It is important that the skin is well hydrated, preventing loss of moisture and promoting skin integrity to minimise the risk of infection entering the body. The effect of sun on the skin has increased moisture loss and damaged the skin. Rob is at increased risk of infection because his skin is now dry and flaky.

Rob needs to act now to prevent further skin damage and potential problems with infection. He is reluctant to use greasy creams and may also be worried that they will have a slight perfume. Although he would benefit from using an emollient ointment for a few days until the skin condition improves, he is likely to be more accepting of an emollient lotion which is less greasy and without perfume. Lotions are easily applied and absorbed into the skin. If he is able to see the benefit of their use, he may be more willing to consider regular use in the future to maintain a healthy condition to his skin. Rob also needs to be reminded about the use of sun protection on future holidays.

Case Scenario 2

Angela is 75 years of age and lives alone. She received treatment for carcinoma of the cervix ten years ago and developed lymphoedema in both legs approximately five years ago. She has been wearing compression stockings to control the swelling but over recent months she has become less mobile and has not been looking after herself very well. Her legs have become very swollen with dry, scaly skin. She has been applying her favourite body cream every few days but the skin is still very dry, with large flakes of skin sticking to her tights and trousers. Recently Angela has noticed a dirty-looking area of skin on her ankle, which she cannot get clean, and the area between her toes has become itchy.

Consider Angela's history and reflect upon why the condition of her skin has deteriorated.

- What skin care advice does Angela need?
- What emollients should she be using and how often?

There are a number of reasons why Angela's skin condition has deteriorated.

1. Angela is less mobile so it is likely that the swelling has increased because of immobility. The capillary filtration rate is raised due to increased venous pressure as the muscle pump remains inactive, with the result that swelling increases in both feet and legs.
2. Increased stasis of lymph fluid will trigger an inflammatory response which leads to a reduction in macrophage activity and an overgrowth of interstitial connective tissue. The delicate physiological balance that maintains integrity of the skin is affected and the skin becomes dehydrated.
3. Angela is not cleansing and moisturising her skin appropriately. Cleansing will remove the build-up of dead skin cells and moisturising will encourage moisture to be retained by the skin and promote skin integrity.

Angela should adopt a twice-daily skin care regime until the condition of her skin improves and she should then continue to cleanse and moisturise her legs every day. She also needs to use an antifungal preparation daily between her toes where it is likely that she has developed tinea pedis (athlete's foot).

Angela should soak her legs in an oily bath emollient and use a soap substitute twice a day to soften the build-up of dead skin cells and assist their removal. After careful drying, a moisturising emollient ointment should be applied to both legs to form an impermeable layer over the skin which will minimise moisture loss and promote skin integrity. The dry, dirty-looking area on her ankle is likely to be the beginning of hyper-keratosis and may require the careful application of salicylic acid if the scales of skin are not loosened by the emollient ointment.

Angela should also be encouraged to take several short walks during the day to promote muscle pump action and a reduction in venous pressure. This in turn will improve lymph drainage.

Conclusion

Care of the skin is important for all patients who have or are at risk of developing lymphoedema. Daily moisturising with an emollient preparation after cleansing will prevent moisture loss and encourage skin integrity.

The development of mild skin conditions, such as dry skin, should be avoided as the colonisation of bacteria that occurs in this condition can increase the risk of infection in a limb where immunity is already compromised, and progression to further more complex problems may result.

All health-care professionals have an important role in educating patients about the care of their skin. Patients can then become informed, active

participants in the adoption of a health-promoting activity aimed at minimising the possibility of future complications.

References

Allen K., Duncan A. and Maguire J. (2004) Patient hygiene. In: L. Dougherty and
   S. Lister (eds) *The Royal Marsden Manual of Clinical Nursing Procedures*, 6th edn.
   Blackwell Publishing, Oxford, pp. 580–6.
Badger C. and Jeffs E. (1995) *Assessment Tool for Assessment of Skin Condition*. Cancer
   Relief Macmillan Fund/University of Manchester/St Catherine's Hospice,
   Crawley.
Board J. and Harlow W. (2002) Lymphoedema 3: the available treatment for
   lymphoedema. *British Journal of Nursing*, **11**(7): 438–50.
British Lymphology Society (BLS) and Lymphoedema Support Network (LSN)
   (2005) *Consensus Document on the Management of Cellulitis in Lymphoedema*. British
   Lymphology Society, Sevenoaks.
Foldi E. and Foldi M. (2003) Lymphostatic diseases. In: M. Foldi, E. Foldi and
   S. Kubik (eds) *Textbook of Lymphology for Physicians and Lymphoedema Therapists*.
   Urban and Fischer, Germany, pp. 232–319.
Keeley V. (2000) Clinical features of lymphoedema. In: R. Twycross, K. Jenns and
   J. Todd (eds) *Lymphoedema*. Radcliffe Medical Press, Oxford, pp. 44–67.
Kumar P. and Clark M. (2005) *Clinical Medicine (MRCP Study Guides)*, 6th edn.
   W.B. Saunders, London.
Linnett N. (2000) Skin management in lymphoedema. In: R. Twycross, K. Jenns and
   J. Todd (eds) *Lymphoedema*. Radcliffe Medical Press, Oxford, pp. 118–29.
Lymphoedema Support Network (LSN) (2006) *Management of Cellulitis in
   Lymphoedema*. Lymphoedema Support Network, London.
Maclaren J. (2001) Skin changes in lymphoedema: pathophysiology and manage-
   ment options. *International Journal of Palliative Nursing*, **7**(8): 381–8.
Marieb E. (2005) Skin and body membranes. In: *Essentials of Human Anatomy and
   Physiology*, 8th edn. Benjamin Cummings, San Francisco.
Masmoudi A., Maaloul I., Turki H. et al. (2005) Erysipelas after breast cancer
   treatment (26 cases). *Dermatology Online Journal*, **11**(3): 12–17. Available at:
   www.dermatology.cdlib.org (accessed 21/3/06).
Mortimer P. (1995) The dermatologist's contribution to lymphoedema management.
   Scope on Phlebology and Lymphology, **2**(3): 17–19.
Mortimer P. (2000) Acute inflammatory episodes. In: R. Twycross, K. Jenns and
   J. Todd (eds) *Lymphoedema*. Radcliffe Medical Press, Oxford, pp. 130–9.
Penzer R. (2003) Lymphoedema. *Nursing Standard*, **17**(35): 45–52.
Williams A. and Venables J. (1996) Skin care in patients with uncomplicated
   lymphoedema. *Journal of Wound Care*, **5**(5): 223–6.
Woo P., Lum P., Wong S., Cheng V. and Yuen K. (2000) Cellulitis complicating
   lymphoedema. *European Journal of Clinical Microbiological Infectious Diseases*,
   19(4): 294–7.

7 Movement and Exercise

Introduction

Body movement is a complex phenomenon, essential for health. Voluntary and involuntary movements take place continuously throughout the body to ensure that it functions in an efficient and effective manner for health to be maintained.

Body movement which uses energy is termed physical activity or exercise (Mullen 2005) and is widely regarded as beneficial for health and well-being. In the care of the patient with, or at risk of, lymphoedema, a regular, gentle exercise regime is thought to enhance lymph drainage and promote a full range of movement in the joints (Hughes 2000, McKenzie 1998, Miller 1996). Overuse or excessive exertion of a limb is thought to increase lymphoedema or induce its development in the patient at risk (Harris & Niesen-Vertommen 2000, Jenns 2000).

Regaining a full range of movement following irradiation or surgical treatment in lymph node areas can be problematic for some due to discomfort and stiffness. As the movement of lymphatic fluid is influenced by muscular activity, any reduction in limb movement can cause a reduction in lymph drainage from the limb.

This chapter will explore the role of movement and exercise in the management of lymphoedema to enable the health-care professional to consider its value with individual patients and to assist with the provision of appropriate advice.

Learning objectives

At the end of this chapter the reader will be able to:

- describe the physiological and psychological effects of exercise

Table 7.1   The effect of exercise (adapted from Hughes 2000).

Arterial supply	Venous return
The arteries supply nutrients and oxygen to the body	60% of the blood is in the venous circulation, which acts as a reservoir for storing blood.
Increased muscular activity demands more oxygen and nutrients from the arteries	The deep transport veins in the muscles respond to muscular activity.
As arterial demand increases with exercise, arterial blood is diverted to skeletal muscle and the heart beats faster	The perforating veins passing through connective tissue are compressed by muscular activity.
Lymph formation is proportional to arterial flow	The valves determine the direction of venous return, allowing blood to flow only in the direction of the heart.
Vigorous activity leads to increased lymph production	Venous return is improved by muscle activity.

- discuss the value of movement and exercise upon lymphatic function in lymphoedema management
- demonstrate knowledge regarding the use of movement and exercise to be able to advise patients with, or at risk of, lymphoedema about a suitable, simple, appropriate exercise regime.

The physiological effects of exercise

Exercise has a direct effect upon the circulation of the body, influencing the arteries and venous return. Table 7.1 summarises these effects but the key physiological effects of exercise are considered to be:

- an increase in cellular metabolism
- an increase in blood pressure
- an increase in respiratory rate
- an enhancement of the body's immune system.

Regular physical exercise can lead to a healthy lifestyle with improved physical fitness and it can also delay death and assist in the avoidance of disease. Benefits include:

- the maintenance of flexible joints and improved muscle function to decrease symptoms of arthritis (Mullen 2005)

- the promotion of new bone formation and the delay of bone loss which helps to decrease the risk of osteoporosis (Nelson et al. 1994)
- an improvement in heart and circulatory function to decrease the risk of heart disease (Box 2004)
- the control of blood pressure to decrease the risk of heart disease and strokes (Box 2004)
- the maintenance of body weight by decreasing body fat (Dunn et al. 1999)
- a reduction in mental and muscular tension which leads to improved concentration and energy levels (Mullen 2005).

The psychological effects of exercise

Exercise can also have a profound effect upon feelings of well-being and even short bursts of activity can be beneficial. Studies have shown that exercise can:

- improve mood (Hansen et al. 2001)
- decrease moderate depression (Salmon 2001)
- reduce anxiety and stress (Hassmen et al. 2000)
- enhance self-esteem and social integration (Hassmen et al. 2000).

In psychological conditions such as depression, exercise alone will not produce improvement but should be viewed as a factor involved in facilitating an enhancement in psychological well-being. Exercise can be fun and encourage people to think differently about themselves.

Movement, function and exercise in lymphoedema

Patients with lymphoedema of the arm following treatment for breast cancer can experience stiffness in their shoulder. Johansson et al. (2001) observed that a decrease in shoulder mobility can develop one month after surgery for breast cancer whilst Tengrup et al. (2001) noted that shoulder discomfort was still being experienced by some patients five years after breast surgery. There is no research to indicate the effect of pelvic surgery and radiotherapy to the major lymph nodes of the inguinal region upon function, but it is possible that similar problems may occur.

Hughes (2000) suggests that the action of the muscle pump during exercise improves lymph drainage. The uptake of lymph and its movement into the collecting and transporting vessels are dependent upon limb movement and muscle contraction, which propel the lymph towards the collecting vessels from where it can be drained. The transport of lymph is also dependent upon movement between the skin and the underlying tissues, so activity of the muscles involving movement of the skin will enhance lymph drainage (Hughes 2000).

Casley-Smith (2001) suggests that a specific order of exercises is required to promote lymph drainage from a limb. The clearing of a drainage reservoir for the lymph fluid is carried out first using massage and then specific exercises are designed to promote lymph drainage into the cleared area. The exercises are combined with relaxation to allow maximum lymph drainage and the addition of breathing exercises increases intrathoracic pressure and assists the pumping of the deep lymphatics. Casley-Smith's approach to exercise is similar to the sequence of movements used by a therapist performing manual lymph drainage. Rhythm and tempo are considered important during completion of the exercises which take 30 minutes to complete and are followed by 30 minutes of relaxation (Casley-Smith 2001).

Although additional specific exercises may be of value in lymphoedema management, particularly when function has been reduced, all limb movement is crucial to promote lymph drainage. Patients with lymphoedema and those at risk of its development need advice concerning the impact of different types of movement and exercises completed in their daily life to understand which ones are beneficial and which ones are not. Many patients already follow an exercise regime or participate in hobbies or activities of a physical nature. Knowledge of how these can be incorporated into their life is essential if patients are to successfully control their swelling or minimise the risk of its development.

Movement and exercise of the limb should be carried out to:

- promote lymph drainage from the limb
- maintain or improve the range of movement of the limb
- strengthen the limb and rebuild muscle tone
- enhance the patient's well-being.

Muscular activity

Movement can be carried out actively by the patient in a free, assisted or resisted manner or passively using mechanical means or with assistance from another patient.

When advising a patient concerning any physical activity, some understanding of the different types of muscle activity and muscle work is important.

- Isotonic exercises involve contraction of the muscle as it is lengthened or shortened. An increase in intramuscular tension occurs at the beginning and end of each exercise. An example of this type of exercise is the use of free weights or exercises carried out against a fixed resistance but caution should be advised as there may be an uneven force throughout each exercise.

- Isometric exercises involve contraction of the muscle as it remains unchanged in length and an increase in intramuscular tension occurs as force is applied against a resistant object. An example of this type of activity would be pushing against a brick wall where there is tension in the muscles but no movement.
- Static muscle work involves a constant muscle contraction to counterbalance opposing forces without producing any movement in the muscle. Examples of this type of activity include pushing or carrying a heavy load and holding a weight away from the body. Static muscle work should not be prolonged as it leads to muscle fatigue. Excessive static muscle work, repeated over time, can lead to joint and ligament damage.
- Eccentric muscle work involves passive contraction of the muscle which lengthens as it opposes the force of a weight. An example of this type of activity would be walking down stairs or lowering an article or load where movement is in the opposite direction to muscle pull.
- Concentric muscle work involves active contraction of the muscle which shortens to produce movement. An example of this is stepping upwards or completing knee raises.

Exercise advice for patients

In order to encourage the patient to recognise the importance of an exercise programme and become compliant in its completion, the health-care professional should consider the patient's lifestyle, goals and hobbies to make sure that what is discussed is relevant and will fit into their daily life.

Muscles work together in groups to ensure that all movement is controlled (Hughes 2000). The deeper muscles provide stability for the body as the superficial muscles produce the required movement. Ideal activities for patients with, or at risk of, lymphoedema are those that involve a combination of muscle activity within the patient's range of movement and ability. Table 7.2 outlines advice for patients to follow concerning exercise and activities.

The effect of vigorous activity and exercise

Patients with, or at risk of, lymphoedema should understand the potential impact of vigorous activity or repetitive exercises upon their limb in order to recognise any implications that may occur following inappropriate activity.

Table 7.2   Advice to patients with or at risk of lymphoedema.

What type of exercise is advisable?	A variety of isotonic and isometric muscle work is advised: ● Swimming ● Cycling ● Walking ● Gentle aerobic/aqua aerobic exercises.
How often?	A graduated programme of exercise which builds upon ability and developing fitness. Some form of exercise completed daily is advantageous.
How vigorous?	A moderate rather than strenuous level. Muscle fatigue, pain and stiffness should not be experienced. Activity should be slow and rhythmical followed by rest periods.
What activities should be avoided?	Excessive straining or repetitive activities involving static muscle work: ● Arm swelling: heavy lifting, carrying, pulling or pushing. Prolonged keyboard work, knitting and writing for long periods. ● Leg swelling: prolonged standing in one position or sitting with legs down. Long journeys without regular breaks to enable movement.
What about previously completed sports?	Sport participation should be built up gradually, assessing the impact upon the limb as activity increases. If muscle fatigue, pain or stiffness occurs, caution should be applied.

Strenuous or vigorous activity is thought to cause an increase in blood supply and capillary filtration rate, with a subsequent increase in lymph production (Hughes 2000). There is therefore the potential for swelling to accumulate where lymph drainage is reduced. If the body is subjected to excessive or unusual activity, there is also the possibility that trauma may occur in the tissues or muscles, causing an inflammatory reaction and the production of more lymph fluid.

Harris & Niesen-Vertommen (2000), in a study of women competing in dragon boat racing, challenged the view that vigorous exercise may be a factor in the development of lymphoedema, and other studies (McKenzie & Kalda 2003, Turner et al. 2004) have observed the effects of breast cancer patients undergoing controlled but moderately intensive exercise regimes. The findings of these studies suggest that arm circumference and arm volume are not influenced by activities of a more exertive nature when carried out by women at risk of lymphoedema. However, it is not known how long-term exercise of this nature affects the lymphatic system and care should be taken to consider an appropriate exercise regime for the individual patient, building up tolerance to exercise slowly and gently.

Limb elevation

Elevation of a swollen limb when at rest is sometimes considered helpful in reducing lymphoedema, particularly if the swollen limb is raised to the level of the heart. Hughes (2000) suggests that in this position, lymphatic and venous drainage are maximised.

Arm elevation should not exceed shoulder height as this can obstruct venous return from the arm. A suitable, comfortable position can be achieved with the swollen arm resting on a pillow placed on the arm of the chair.

The ideal position for leg elevation is with the body horizontal. The legs can be supported on a pillow but it is important to ensure that they are not raised higher than the head so that venous drainage from the head and neck is not reduced. Legs can be supported on a stool when sitting.

Simple arm and shoulder exercises

The following simple exercises will encourage lymph drainage from the arm and promote shoulder movement. If the patient wears a compression garment, this should be worn as the exercises are completed. The exercises can be performed daily but if the arm begins to ache during the exercise, it is important to reduce the activity. Additional advice may be required from a physiotherapist if difficulties occur. The arm should be in a comfortable position, resting on a pillow which has been placed on the arm of the chair or the patient's knee.

- Slowly make a tight fist and then spread the fingers out wide. Repeat ten times.
- With the palm of the hand facing down, slowly flex the wrist upwards and then back down again to point the fingers to the floor. Repeat ten times.
- With the arm straight and the palm facing upwards towards the ceiling, slowly bend the forearm up to touch the shoulder and then slowly straighten again. Repeat ten times.
- With the hand behind the body, reach up the back as far as possible without causing discomfort.
- With the head held still, lift the arm to place the hand behind the head.

Simple leg exercises

The following simple exercises will encourage lymph drainage from the leg and help to keep the joints mobile. Whenever possible, they should be combined with regular walking, swimming or cycling within the patient's capabilities. If the patient wears a compression garment, this should be worn during all exercises, except those in water. The exercises can be completed twice daily and should be followed by a short rest. If the leg begins to ache, the activity should be reduced.

- Bend and stretch the toes up and down for a slow count to ten.
- Flex the foot up and down at the ankle for a slow count to ten.
- Make slow, rhythmical circles with the foot for a slow count to ten.
- Bend and stretch the knee in a controlled, slow movement.

The following case scenarios illustrate the role of appropriate exercise in the management of lymphoedema.

Case Scenario 1

Jessica is a 40-year-old aerobics teacher who six months ago underwent a simple mastectomy for breast cancer. Being aware of the risk of lymphoedema developing in her arm following the surgery, Jessica closely followed the advice she was given by her breast care nurse. She reduced the number of classes she was teaching each week by half and carefully looked after her skin. Her intention was to build up the number of aerobic classes she taught again slowly but in the meantime, she started some gentle yoga exercises and went to the gym a few times each week to ensure that she maintained her fitness level. She was disappointed to find that some swelling developed around her forearm and elbow some months later. She tells you that her yoga exercises involve floor work where she uses her arms to support her body and that at the gym she has been using the rowing machine and treadmill.

   Consider Jessica's history and reflect upon possible factors involved in the appearance of the swelling.

- Why do you think Jessica has developed arm swelling?
- Do you think she needs to increase, reduce or change her exercise regime?
- How would you advise Jessica regarding the type of exercises she should carry out with her arm?

Jessica is at risk of developing lymphoedema in her arm following surgery for breast cancer when some of the lymph nodes in her axilla will have been surgically removed. Jessica was sensible to reduce the number of aerobic classes she held after her surgery in order to build up her ability to tolerate these classes again slowly. However, the alternative exercises she has been completing appear to have been too exertive for her arm.

Although she does not need to reduce her activity further, Jessica should concentrate on yoga exercises which do not require her to put weight through her arms. The isometric muscle activity required to support her body weight during the yoga exercises she has been doing involve static muscle work and excessive straining. This can lead to the development of lymphoedema in an at-risk limb.

Jessica also needs to modify her gym work and avoid the use of the rowing machine where eccentric muscle work involves repetitive movements. These can lead to muscle strain and the development of lymphoedema if the repetition is prolonged.

There is no reason why Jessica's fitness level should reduce because of her breast cancer treatment. She can continue to teach aerobics and slowly increase the number of classes she holds. In the meantime some modification to her yoga and gym exercises is required and she may like to consider the addition of swimming to her exercise regime which involves a variety of isotonic and isometric exercises.

Case Scenario 2

Sam and his wife Lil enjoy ballroom dancing on a regular twice-weekly basis and are proud of their achievements in competitive events. At 75 years of age, they have enjoyed good health despite Sam's treatment for non-Hodgkin's lymphoma five years ago. Sam developed some lymphoedema in his leg following the surgery to his groin nodes, but he wears a compression stocking and is thankful that the swelling is well controlled. He has not experienced any problems with his leg since he started wearing the compression stocking.

Three months ago Lil suffered a mild stroke which left her with a weakness on her right side. Sam has been caring for his wife and has rarely left the house because he does not want to leave his wife alone. They have good neighbours who have helped with the shopping. Recently Sam noticed that his leg swelling had increased and that his stocking was becoming tight. Thinking that his stocking was due to be replaced, he asked for another and mentioned that he had become concerned about the increased swelling.

Consider Sam's history and reflect upon possible factors that may cause his leg swelling to worsen.

- Why do you think Sam's leg swelling may have increased?
- Do you think he needs to increase, reduce or change his exercise regime?

- How would you advise Sam regarding the type of exercises he should complete?

Although Sam's leg swelling has been well controlled for the past five years, any significant change should be investigated to ensure that there is no recurrence of disease causing an obstruction within the remaining lymph nodes. The possibility of infection should also be considered and explored by closely examining the leg for signs of inflammation.

As Lil has been ill for some months, Sam's regular activities have undergone a change. He has become relatively housebound whilst looking after Lil and this reduction in activity is likely to have had an impact upon his leg swelling. Regular ballroom dancing every week involving isotonic and isometric muscle work, combined with a compression stocking and an active life, have enabled Sam to keep good control of his leg swelling until now. As this changed when Lil became ill, Sam now needs to consider alternative ways of increasing his activity. It may be possible for a neighbour to sit with Lil while Sam does the shopping or takes a daily walk. Alternatively, he could take Lil for a walk in a wheelchair until she feels able to walk safely again and build up her strength. A stronger compression stocking could also be considered if this is appropriate in order to provide more compression to the leg if the swelling has increased. Combined with some activity, increased compression should help to reduce the swelling. If Sam and Lil are able to return to their ballroom dancing, the problem may fully resolve but until then Sam needs to ensure that his activity levels match those that he previously enjoyed in order to control his leg swelling.

Conclusion

Regular movement and exercise hold many benefits for health and well-being. In the patient with lymphoedema, gentle regular exercise increases lymph flow and reduces the risk of fluid accumulating. By incorporating movement and exercise into a self-care programme of lymphoedema management, the patient is encouraged to focus on what can be achieved within a normal, active lifestyle into which activities previously enjoyed can be incorporated.

References

Box R. (2004) Exercise and lymphoedema. *Swell News. Lymphoedema Association of Victoria*, **57**: 1–7.

Casley-Smith J. (2001) Exercises for lymphoedema. *British Lymphology Society Newsletter*, **30**: 16–18.

Dunn A., Marcus B., Kampert J., Garcia M., Kohl H. and Blair S. (1999) Comparisons of lifestyle and structured interventions to increase physical activity and cardiovascular fitness: a randomised control trial. *Journal of the American Medical Association*, **281**(4): 327–34.

Hansen C., Stevens L. and Coast J. (2001) Exercise duration and mood state: how much is enough to feel better? *Health Psychology*, **20**(4): 267–75.

Harris S. and Niesen-Vertommen S. (2000) Challenging the myth of exercise induced lymphoedema following breast cancer: a series of case reports. *Journal of Surgical Oncology*, **74**(2): 95–9.

Hassmen P., Koivula N. and Uutela A. (2000) Physical exercise and psychological well-being: a population study in Finland. *Preventive Medicine*, **30**(1): 17–25.

Hughes K. (2000) Exercise and lymphoedema. In: R. Twycross, K. Jenns and J. Todd (eds) *Lymphoedema*. Radcliffe Medical Press, Oxford, pp. 140–64.

Jenns K. (2000) Management strategies. In: R. Twycross, K. Jenns and J. Todd (eds) *Lymphoedema*. Radcliffe Medical Press, Oxford, pp. 97–117.

Johansson K., Ingvar C., Albertson M. and Ekdahl C. (2001) Arm lymphoedema, shoulder mobility and muscle strength after breast cancer treatment. *Advances in Physiotherapy*, **3**(2): 55–66.

McKenzie D. (1998) Abreast in a boat. *Canadian Medical Association Journal*, **159**(4): 376–8.

McKenzie D. and Kalda A. (2003) Effect of upper extremity exercise on secondary lymphoedema in breast cancer patients: a pilot study. *Journal of Clinical Oncology*, **21**(3): 463–6.

Miller L. (1996) The enigma of exercise. National Lymphoedema Network Newsletter, Oct–Dec: 15–16.

Mullen D. (2005) The benefits of exercise. Spine Universe Newsletter for Patients, St Louis. www.spinenewsletter.com (accessed 17/4/07).

Nelson M., Fiatarone M., Morganti C., Trice I., Greenberg R. and Evans W. (1994) Effects of high-intensity strength training on multiple risk factors for osteoporotic fractures. A randomised controlled trial. *Journal of the American Medical Association*, **272**(24): 1909–14.

Salmon P. (2001) Effects of physical exercise on anxiety, depression and sensitivity to stress: a unifying theory. *Clinical Psychology Review*, **21**(1): 33–61.

Tengrup I., Tennvall-Nittby L., Christiansson I. and Laurin M. (2001) Arm morbidity after breast conserving therapy for breast cancer. *Acta Oncologica*, **39**(3): 393–7.

Turner J., Hayes S. and Reul-Hirche H. (2004) Improving the physical status and quality of life of women treated for breast cancer: a pilot study of a structured exercise intervention. *Journal of Surgical Oncology*, **86**(3): 141–6.

8 Lymphatic Drainage

Introduction

In order to understand the role of lymphatic drainage massage in the management of lymphoedema, a brief revision of the lymphatic system is required.

The initial lymphatics are positioned just under the surface of the skin and are composed of a very thin, delicate structure, one cell thick. Lymph fluid enters the initial lymphatic from the interstitial compartment of the tissues and moves towards the lymph drainage channels, aided by muscular contractions, arterial pulsations, deep diaphragmatic breathing and contraction of the intestines during digestion (Stanton 2000). In a healthy lymph system, lymph fluid is then constantly filtered throughout the lymph system via valvular vessels which rhythmically contract and relax. If the lymphatic system has become altered, either following intervention or because of an abnormality, the available drainage routes for lymph fluid are reduced and those that remain can quickly become overloaded.

The opening of the initial lymphatics and drainage of lymph fluid can be encouraged by gentle massage movements performed on the skin. This increases activity within the lymphatics so that the lymph channels drain more effectively and lymph fluid is encouraged to move towards the lymph nodes. These specialised massage movements are performed by a specially trained therapist in areas of the body where lymph drainage is altered but the movements can be adapted so that they can be performed by the patient in areas of the body where there is normal lymph drainage.

The aim of this chapter is to outline the two types of lymphatic drainage used in the management of lymphoedema:

- manual lymphatic drainage (MLD), performed by a trained therapist
- simple lymphatic drainage (SLD), performed by the patient.

Learning objectives

At the end of this chapter the reader will be able to:

- outline the background to MLD and SLD
- describe the aims and basic principles of MLD and SLD
- discuss the use of MLD and SLD in the management of lymphoedema
- identify circumstances where MLD and SLD should not be used.

Manual lymphatic drainage

Background

The history of the technique termed MLD can be traced back to the 1930s when it was developed in Europe by Dr Emil Vodder, following extensive research into the lymph system. The early massage movements of the skin developed from this research were used to treat a variety of acute conditions where swelling was present, with positive benefits observed (Wittlinger & Wittlinger 1990).

During the next 30 years, the technique grew within the field of alternative and complementary therapy where it was used to treat acute and chronic inflammations of a surgical, dermatological, neurological and musculoskeletal nature, plus circulatory disturbances and for the reduction of stress (MLD UK 2001, Nickalls 1996). Then in the 1960s the role of MLD was reviewed, adjusted and improved by a German physician, Földi, and a Belgian physician, Leduc, to facilitate its use among patients with lymphostatic disease (Derdeyrn et al. 1993). A number of schools of MLD therapy, illustrated in Table 8.1, have subsequently evolved, with differences between them focused primarily on the sequence of hand movements used. However, the general approach to MLD remains very similar and many MLD therapists use a blend of approaches when treating patients with MLD.

The aim of MLD

The primary aim of MLD is to improve the functioning of the lymphatic system. A series of pumping and stretching hand movements in a range of sequences are used to move the skin in specific directions based on the underlying structure and physiology of the lymphatic system. The movements influence the lymph vessels which transport lymph towards the lymph nodes.

Where lymphoedema is present, MLD can be used as an aspect of treatment in combination with other approaches to management of the swelling.

Table 8.1   MLD training schools.

Vodder in Austria
Foldi in Germany
Leduc in Belgium
Casley-Smith in Australia

Its aim is to increase activity within the normal lymphatics so that lymph drains more effectively within them, bypassing the damaged or obstructed lymph channels and transferring lymph across 'watersheds' into adjacent areas of the body where it can drain more easily (Tribe 1995).

The aims of MLD are therefore to:

● increase activity in normal lymphatics and improve their function
● open the flow of lymph fluid across watersheds
● encourage lymph fluid to flow along alternative drainage routes
● aid lymph drainage from congested areas.

The basic principles of MLD

In order to move fluid from a swollen area towards functioning lymphatics, the movements start at the neck and unaffected lymphatics first, then move towards the area of the trunk closest to the affected area before finally being completed on the swollen area itself. Figure 8.1 shows MLD being completed on the trunk.

Lymphatic drainage movements are based on the principle of motion. The initial lymphatics are opened up by a straight motion performed with light pressure on the skin in order to stretch it gently, followed by a lateral motion to stimulate the initial lymphatics to drain. The initial lymphatics then need to close to ensure that the lymph drains, so the pressure is released and the stretched skin springs back to its normal position (Strossenreuther 2003).

There are four different techniques used in MLD.

● Stationary circles
● Rotary technique
● Pump technique
● Scoop technique

The hand movements required for these different techniques are used according to the area of the body being treated (Wittlinger & Wittlinger 1990) and involve one or both hands in a slow rhythmical repetitive manner (Strossenreuther 2003).

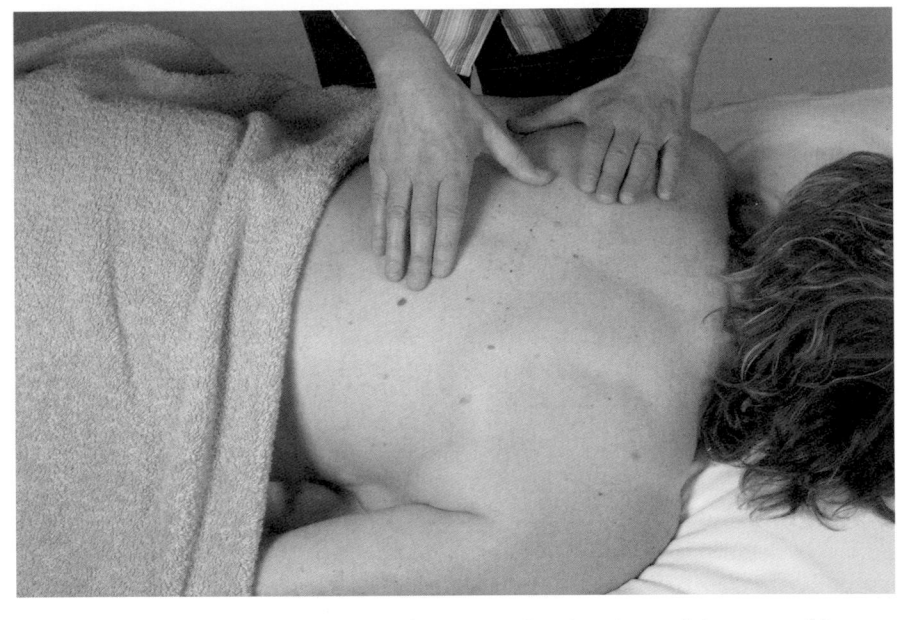

Figure 8.1   Manual lymphatic drainage being completed on the trunk (courtesy of Anne Williams).

For MLD to be completed correctly, a trained therapist will ensure that:

- the correct pressure is used on the skin. If the pressure used is too deep, the initial lymphatics may become damaged or collapse so that drainage does not occur. If the pressure is too light, the fingers will slide over the skin
- the movements are completed slowly, rhythmically and repetitively. Lymph can be compared with honey which takes time to move (Wittlinger & Wittlinger 1990). If the movements are completed too quickly, there is insufficient time for the initial lymphatics to open, drain and close again
- an appropriate sequence and number of movements are used to direct the lymph fluid towards the appropriate lymph nodes. By clearing the way ahead, a path is created for the lymph fluid to flow along, so MLD movements are always started close to the node to encourage the lymph fluid to flow there.

Treatment with MLD

MLD requires a 'hands-on' approach where the patient becomes dependent upon the skills of the therapist. It is labour intensive with no guarantees regarding the outcome and the most frequently used model of treatment requires patients to undergo a three-week course of one hour per day.

During the treatment sessions, the patient is encouraged to relax and following completion of the treatment, a simplified form of self-massage is usually taught for the patient to continue independently. Regular follow-up sessions of MLD may occur at weekly or monthly intervals to maintain lymph drainage.

MLD is usually provided by trained therapists on a fee-paying basis.

The use of MLD in the management of lymphoedema

As an aspect of treatment for lymphoedema, MLD is not considered beneficial when used in isolation (Andersen et al. 2000, Foldi 1998, Leduc et al. 1998, Mortimer 2003). Studies carried out in Europe support its place within a combination of treatments to reduce limb volume over a short, specified period of time (Johansson et al. 1999, Piller et al. 1993) but the long-term outcomes of treatment using MLD are not known.

In a randomised crossover trial by Williams et al. (2002) comparing the use of compression hosiery with or without MLD, a number of effects were attributed to the use of MLD. These included improved quality of life, a greater reduction in arm volume and a reduction in skin thickness. The study was limited to patients with breast cancer-related lymphoedema of one arm, but suggested that the effects of MLD may be greater than just limb volume reduction.

In a qualitative study carried out by Woods (2003), patients with lymphoedema who had undergone a course of treatment with MLD observed an improvement in the physical symptoms they associated with their lymphoedema. MLD was also reported to induce relaxation through touch and it is possible that this is necessary for lymph to drain as the treatment is given (Woods 2003).

MLD is frequently used during the intensive phase of lymphoedema management in combination with other aspects of treatment. However, it is also used in the following circumstances:

- lymphoedema of the face, neck, genitals, breast and abdominal areas
- trunk and midline lymphoedema.

There is no evidence to suggest that MLD is a useful treatment for patients at risk of developing lymphoedema in order to prevent its occurrence.

When MLD should not be used

There are some circumstances in which the use of MLD is not advisable.

- *Acute infection or inflammation.* MLD may cause pain or discomfort if infection or inflammation is present in the area to be treated. In addition, toxic substances may be moved into lymph channels and spread throughout the body rather than being eliminated by the action of the local lymph nodes.

- *Active, untreated malignant disease*. Concern exists that MLD may encourage the transport of cancer cells in untreated active disease (Wittlinger & Wittlinger 1990).
- *Recent thrombosis*. Until anticoagulation therapy is well established, there is a risk of clot dislodgement if MLD is carried out in an area where a thrombosis is known to have developed.
- *Cardiac oedema*. If the heart is not fully functioning, there is a risk of cardiac overload as a result of MLD treatment.

Simple lymphatic drainage (SLD)

Background

SLD is based on the principles of MLD. The hand movements are simplified and the technique modified to enable patients to incorporate an easier technique of lymphatic drainage into the daily management of their lymphoedema. SLD can be particularly useful when the more specialised skills of an MLD therapist are not available or when the patient has completed a course of intensive therapy to reduce their swelling. It is used in conjunction with other aspects of lymphoedema management and not in isolation.

SLD is widely recognised as an aspect of lymphoedema management in the UK and there are anecdotal reports of perceived benefits obtained from its daily use within a self-care regime of lymphoedema management.

The aim of SLD

The main aim of SLD is to provide a modified technique of MLD that the patient can complete independently of a therapist (BLS 2001). It aims to:

- stimulate normal draining lymphatics
- encourage lymph fluid to move away from congested areas to areas where it can drain away more freely
- improve superficial lymph drainage.

The basic principles of SLD

SLD is completed in areas where lymph drainage is unaffected by any treatment intervention or altered lymph drainage pattern. This means that areas that are swollen are not included in the technique because lymphatic massage in these areas requires the skill of a trained MLD therapist to ensure that lymph fluid is moved in the correct direction. By working on areas where lymph drainage is believed to be normal, SLD can encourage lymph fluid to move from the swollen area to areas where it can drain away more easily by clearing the route ahead.

The technique can be likened to road works on a busy road. In order to bypass the road works, the traffic has to find alternative routes around the obstruction. These alternative, minor routes, already working hard to keep local traffic moving, can quickly become congested unless the traffic is allowed to flow freely. So by ensuring that there are no obstacles in the way, the routes are able to cope with the increase in traffic and the congestion is eased.

The hand movements used in SLD are simplified versions of those used in MLD which follow a set sequence to encourage lymph fluid to drain.

Treatment with SLD

SLD is a patient-led aspect of lymphoedema management taught by the therapist for the patient to use independently. It can be used once or twice daily, depending upon the patient's wishes, and completion of the full technique should take about 20 minutes.

There are some important points that need to be considered prior to completion of the technique.

- The patient should choose a quiet time with no disturbances. Some patients find it useful to set aside some time as they go to bed to perform the technique as it can be relaxing. Others find it better to perform the technique before they get up in the morning. Whatever the preference, the technique should be fully completed each time.
- The pressure on the skin must be very light. It is important to move the skin only and not the tissues below. If the pressure is too heavy, the skin becomes reddened as blood flows to the surface and if the pressure is too light, the hand slides over the skin rather than remaining in contact with it.
- The technique must be completed in a slow, rhythmical manner. Lymph, like honey, takes time to move and needs to be encouraged.
- Relaxed hands and flat fingers are necessary throughout the technique to ensure that the fingers do not dig into the skin and redden it.
- The use of creams, oil or powder should be avoided in areas where the technique is being carried out to ensure that good contact between the hands and the skin can be maintained.

The use of SLD in the management of lymphoedema

A randomised trial by Sitzia et al. (2002) considered the effectiveness of MLD and SLD in the management of lymphoedema and concluded that MLD was more effective at reducing limb volume than SLD when used in conjunction with compression bandaging. Other outcome measures such as skin condition, limb mobility and quality of life were not considered and the authors acknowledged that in practice, the SLD technique adopted by a patient may differ from that of the study practitioner (Sitzia et al. 2002).

Bellhouse (2000) suggests that SLD has a useful role in the management of lymphoedema, particularly in the following circumstances:

- following a course of MLD provided by a skilled therapist
- during the maintenance phase of lymphoedema management in conjunction with lymphoedema garments
- in the presence of midline oedema such as truncal, midline, facial or genital oedema (Bellhouse 2000, BLS 2001).

Many patients can use SLD in the management of their lymphoedema but in an audit of patients' technique of SLD in the management of lymphoedema, Woods (2001) found that many patients lacked confidence in their ability to undertake this aspect of self-care and were unsure of the benefit it may provide. In addition, many rushed the sequence of movements and made errors in their technique.

Williams et al. (2002) also highlighted difficulties teaching patients the technique of SLD and suggested that the patient's understanding of the movements on the skin and the pressure required was greatly enhanced if they had previously experienced MLD.

A number of other factors should be considered.

- Impaired mobility or function of the upper limbs will make completion of the technique difficult. A relative or friend may be able to help, but it is difficult to achieve the correct pressure on the skin of someone else and may not be acceptable to the patient.
- Poor motivation or compliance may lead to a rushed and inaccurate use of the technique and a possible worsening of the swelling. If a patient is poorly motivated to undertake or continue the technique, it is better to stop.
- The skill and motivation of the patient to complete the technique will be greatly influenced by the quality of the teaching they receive from the therapist. Careful choice of timing to ensure that the patient is receptive to an explanation and demonstration of the technique should be supported by an approach that is sensitive to the patient's needs. Written information should be provided to support the verbal information given.

- The therapist should receive appropriate training in the technique to ensure that they are skilled and confident to teach patients.

When SLD should not be used

SLD is not advisable in the following circumstances which also apply to MLD.

- *Acute infection or inflammation.* SLD may cause pain or discomfort if infection or inflammation is present in the area to be treated. In addition, toxic substances may be moved into lymph channels and spread throughout the body rather than being eliminated by the action of the local lymph nodes.
- *Active, untreated malignant disease.* Concern exists that SLD may encourage the transport of cancer cells in untreated active disease.
- *Recent thrombosis.* Until anticoagulation therapy is well established, it is advisable to avoid SLD in an area where a thrombosis is known to have developed.
- *Cardiac oedema.* If the heart is not fully functioning, there may be a risk of cardiac overload if SLD is regularly carried out.

In addition, SLD should not be carried out if the patient has impaired upper limb function or is poorly motivated to complete the technique.

The following case scenario outlines considerations for the use of MLD in lymphoedema management.

Case Scenario

Pamela is a 47-year-old lady who completed treatment for cervical cancer five years ago. She recently attended a rock festival with her family where she stood for long periods listening to the music and when she returned home she noticed that her right calf was swollen. Her doctor advised her that she had developed lymphoedema.

The swelling is mild, only focused below the knee, and Pamela has noticed that it tends to be worse at the end of the day. She is well and disease free, but very anxious about the swelling because it is visible and stops her from wearing some of her clothes and boots. She has looked for information about lymphoedema on the internet and found out that 'massage' to her leg will help. She asks you to tell her more about the use of massage in the management of lymphoedema and where she can find a massage therapist to treat her leg.

Consider Pamela's history and reflect upon the different aspects of lymphoedema management.

- Do you think 'massage' will help her?
- How would you advise her further?

Pamela should be advised that the type of massage used in the management of lymphoedema is not traditional massage. Deep therapeutic massage used to release muscle tension and help with relaxation is not appropriate in the management of lymphoedema.

Lymphatic drainage is sometimes called 'lymph drainage massage' and Pamela should be made aware that this type of treatment requires a therapist who is skilled in its use with patients who have lymphoedema. A therapist who uses lymphatic drainage in beauty therapy or to manage oedema may not have sufficient training to treat patients who have lymphoedema and altered lymph drainage.

Although lymphatic drainage can be useful in treating Pamela's lymphoedema, the chosen approach of MLD or SLD should always be utilised in conjunction with other aspects of treatment. If the swelling is mild and uncomplicated, Pamela could consider incorporating SLD into the daily management of her swelling once she has received appropriate information and a demonstration of the technique from a skilled therapist. Alternatively, an initial course of MLD from a trained therapist will enable her to continue the simplified version of the technique independently, with a greater understanding of the skin pressure to be used.

Conclusion

Lymphatic drainage has a valuable role in the management of lymphoedema when used in combination with other aspects of treatment. MLD as a therapist-led treatment is primarily used when swelling is complex, whilst the simplified version, SLD, promotes patient independence and can be particularly useful when swelling is mild and uncomplicated.

MLD is popular with patients but a course of treatment may not easily be available and be costly to undertake. The long-term benefits of this aspect of treatment are unknown and require further exploration to firmly secure the place of MLD in the management of lymphoedema.

References

Andersen L., Hojris I., Erlandsen M. and Andersen J. (2000) Treatment of breast-cancer related lymphoedema with or without manual lymphatic drainage. *Acta Oncologica*, **39**(3): 399–405.

Bellhouse S. (2000) Simple lymphatic drainage In: R. Twycross, K. Jenns and J. Todd (eds) *Lymphoedema*. Radcliffe Medical Press, Oxford, pp. 217–35.

British Lymphology Society (BLS) (2001) *Guidelines for the Use of Manual Lymphatic Drainage and Simple Lymphatic Drainage in Lymphoedema.* British Lymphology Society, Sevenoaks.

Derdeyrn A., Aslam P. and Pflug J. (1993) Manual lymph drainage – mode of action. Progress in Lymphology XIV: Proceedings of the 14th International Congress of Lymphology, Washington DC, September 20–26. Eds E.M. Witte and C.L.Witte.

Foldi E. (1998) The treatment of lymphoedema. *Cancer* (supplement), **83**(12): 2833–4.

Johansson K., Albertsson M., Ingvar C. and Ekdahl C. (1999) Effects of compression bandaging with or without manual lymph drainage treatment in patients with postoperative arm lymphoedema. *Lymphology*, **32**(3): 103–10.

Leduc O., Leduc A., Bourgeois P. and Belgrado J. (1998) The physical treatment of upper limb oedema. *Cancer* (supplement), **83**(12): 2835–9.

MLD UK (2001) *Directory of MLD Therapists.* MLD UK, Glenrothes, Scotland. Available at: www.mlduk.org.uk (accessed 26/11/06).

Mortimer P. (2003) Medical and physical treatment. In: N. Browse, K. Burnard and P. Mortimer (eds) *Diseases of the Lymphatics.* Arnold/Oxford University Press, London, pp. 165–78.

Nickalls S. (1996) Fluid forces. *Nursing Times*, **92**(13): 52–3.

Piller N., Swedborg I., Wilking N. and Jensen G. (1993) Short-term manual lymph drainage treatment and maintenance therapy for post-mastectomy lymphoedema. Progress in Lymphology XIV: Proceedings of the 14th International Congress of Lymphology, Washington DC, September 20–26. Eds E.M. Witte and C.L.Witte.

Sitzia J., Sobrido L. and Harlow W. (2002) Manual lymphatic drainage compared with simple lymphatic drainage in the treatment of post-mastectomy lymphoedema. A pilot, randomised trial. *Physiotherapy*, **88**(2): 99–107.

Stanton A. (2000) How does tissue swelling occur? The physiology and pathophysiology of interstitial fluid formation. In: R. Twycross, K. Jenns and J. Todd (eds) *Lymphoedema.* Radcliffe Medical Press, Oxford, pp. 11–21.

Strossenreuther R. (2003) Practical instructions for therapists – manual lymph drainage according to Dr E. Vodder. In: M. Foldi, E. Foldi and S. Kubik (eds) *Textbook of Lymphology for Physicians and Lymphoedema Therapists.* Urban and Fischer, Germany, pp. 496–511.

Tribe K. (1995) Treatment of lymphoedema: the central importance of manual lymph drainage. *Physiotherapy*, **81**(3): 154–6.

Williams A., Vadgama A., Franks P. and Mortimer P. (2002) A randomised controlled crossover trial of manual lymphatic drainage in women with breast cancer-related lymphoedema. *European Journal of Cancer Care*, **11**(4): 254–61.

Wittlinger H. and Wittlinger G. (1990) *Textbook of Dr Vodder's Manual Lymph Drainage, Vol 1, Basic Course,* 3rd edn. Karl F Haug Publishers, Heidelberg, Germany.

Woods M. (2001) Follow me: an audit of patients' technique of simple lymphatic drainage in lymphoedema management. *BLS Book of Conference Abstracts, Innovations in Practice.* British Lymphology Society, Sevenoaks.

Woods M. (2003) The experience of manual lymph drainage as an aspect of treatment for lymphoedema. *International Journal of Palliative Nursing*, **9**(8): 336–41.

9

The Role of Compression Therapy in the Management of Lymphoedema

Introduction

In order to advise and support a patient with, or at risk of, lymphoedema, the health-care professional has a responsibility to understand when compression therapy is indicated and how it can influence swelling. Compression therapy can be provided in the form of compression garments or low-stretch bandages, with the choice based upon clinical and physical indications established during an assessment of the patient.

A variety of physiological effects involving the venous, lymphatic and arterial systems are initiated by the application of compression and can be manipulated by the type of compression applied, the materials and the application technique used. The results achieved by using an appropriate and safe technique can be dramatic as the limb size and shape become altered over time by the compression therapy applied to the limb. This in turn can have a positive impact upon the patient's psychological and psychosocial well-being.

This chapter will explore the role of compression garments and compression bandages in the management of lymphoedema. Although compression bandages will be discussed in some detail, the main purpose of this chapter is to inform the health-care professional regarding the use of compression garments in the management of mild, uncomplicated lymphoedema as the use of compression bandages is a skilled technique for which specialist skills are required.

Learning objectives

At the end of this chapter the reader will be able to:

- describe the two phases of lymphoedema management and the clinical indications for each
- discuss the physiological effects and principles of compression therapy
- outline indications for the use of compression garments
- complete simple limb measurements required for the selection of the correct size of compression garment
- advise a patient concerning the application, removal and care of their compression garment
- outline indications for the use of multilayer compression bandages
- identify, prepare and support a patient who is to undergo a course of multilayer compression bandaging.

The two phases of lymphoedema management

The management of lymphoedema is frequently divided into two phases: a first intensive or reduction phase of management, requiring specialist intervention, and a second maintenance or self-care phase in which the swelling is controlled without the need for specialist intervention (Todd 2000, Woods 2004).

Terms used to describe the two phases of management can vary and include:

- complex decongestive physical therapy (Foldi 1985)
- complex physical therapy (Mason 1993)
- complex lymphoedema therapy (Boris et al. 1994).

Within both phases of management, a combination of treatments is used. These are illustrated in Table 9.1 which highlights that the use of compression therapy differs significantly between the two phases.

The first, intensive phase of management is a short, planned period of treatment with clear aims outlined, discussed and agreed between the patient and the therapist. Consisting of daily treatment delivered by the therapist for a period of 2–3 weeks, this phase incorporates the specialist interventions of compression bandaging and manual lymph drainage together with the adoption of a good skin care regime and exercise programme.

Indications for the intensive phase of management may include:

- a limb volume greater than 20% of the opposite limb requiring reduction (Badger et al. 2000)
- a limb which has become misshapen due to the degree and extent of lymphoedema (Todd 2000)

Table 9.1   The two phases of lymphoedema management.

Intensive phase	Maintenance phase
A short, planned, therapist-led period of treatment usually consisting of daily treatment over three weeks. Clear indications for this aspect of treatment with specific aims and objectives can be identified at the assessment of the patient.	The self-care aspect of lymphoedema management in which the lymphoedema is controlled long term by the patient with minimal specialist intervention.
Aspects of treatment used: ● Skin care ● Movement and exercise ● Multilayer compression bandaging ● Manual lymph drainage	Aspects of treatment used: ● Skin care ● Movement and exercise ● Compression garments ● Simple lymph drainage
Indications for use: ● Large limbs ● Poor shape ● Fragile skin ● Fibrosis	Indications for use: ● Mild/uncomplicated swelling where there is preservation of the limb shape and skin integrity. ● To maintain improvement achieved through an intensive phase of management.

- the presence of fragile or broken skin on a swollen limb which could be further damaged by the use of compression garments (Jenns 2000)
- the presence of fibrosis in the tissues of a swollen limb which could be softened by the use of compression bandages (Woods 2004).

The second, maintenance or self-care phase of management requires motivation and perseverance from the patient in order to achieve long-term control of the swelling. Essentially a patient-led aspect of management, the maintenance phase requires less specialist intervention with a focus on reassessment and evaluation of progress at regular intervals in order to motivate the patient and identify any complicating factors at an early stage while they can easily be managed.

Indications for the maintenance phase of treatment may include:

- a limb volume less than 20% of the opposite limb provided that the shape of the limb has been preserved and the skin is in good condition (Badger et al. 2000)
- to maintain improvement in limb shape and size achieved through a course of intensive therapy (Woods 2004)
- where lymphoedema is mild and uncomplicated with a normal limb shape (Jenns 2000).

Many patients do not need, or want, to undergo an intensive phase of management for their lymphoedema following their first assessment and manage their swelling independently over a long period of time, using treatment strategies outlined within the maintenance phase of management. If an intensive phase of management is required, this may be planned at a later stage when the patient is able to incorporate the requirements of daily visits for treatment into home and work responsibilities.

A variety of health-care professionals in general or community settings will therefore provide the ongoing health-care needs of the patient with mild uncomplicated lymphoedema in the maintenance phase of lymphoedema management. Knowledge concerning the use of compression therapy is therefore essential to ensure that it remains appropriate for the patient in their care.

The physiological effects of compression therapy

The application of compression to a limb initiates physiological effects within the venous, arterial and lymphatic systems. It also has an effect upon the tissues.

Venous system

During walking, the pump action of the calf muscle increases the flow of blood towards the heart. If high levels of compression are applied to the limb, the diameter of the superficial and deep veins can be reduced with the result that venous flow increases (Partch 2003). A combination of compression and muscular activity results in the most marked increase in venous flow.

Arterial system

High levels of compression can cause tissue ischaemia if a patient has lower limb peripheral arterial occlusive disease. Arterial perfusion can be evaluated by recording the ankle/brachial pressure index (ABPI) using a hand-held Doppler and this is essential before the use of compression if the clinical history and physical assessment of a patient identify suspected arterial insufficiency in the lower limb.

Lymphatic system

Compression therapy applied to a swollen limb opposes fluid filtration from blood capillaries into the tissues, reducing the formation of excess tissue fluid and decreasing lymphatic load. In addition, lymph fluid stagnating in the tissues is encouraged to move through the lymphatic channels by the combined influence of compression therapy, acting as a semi-rigid encasement, and physical exercise as the active muscles work against the compression. This results in an increase in lymph drainage from the tissues.

Physiological effects of compression therapy on the tissues

The use of compression increases blood flow in the microcirculation and has been shown to promote an improvement in general skin perfusion (Partch 2003). For the patient with lymphoedema, the increased blood flow initiated by compression can gradually soften the fibrotic changes that develop within the tissues when lymph drainage becomes reduced and lymph fluid stagnates. As the fibrosis reduces, the tissues resume their normal contour and limb shape is restored.

Contraindications for compression therapy

Compression therapy should not be used in the following situations.

- When the patient has suspected or known arterial disease in the affected, swollen limb.
- If the patient has an acute infection in the swollen limb. Compression therapy can be used once the acute phase has settled if tolerated by the patient.
- During the acute stages of a deep vein thrombosis in the leg. Once anti-coagulation therapy has commenced, the use of compression garments can minimise the development of post-thrombotic syndrome.
- In the presence of severe cardiac oedema (Callum et al. 1997).

The principles of compression therapy

In order to make an informed clinical decision concerning the most suitable type of compression therapy for a patient, consideration of the following physical principles is required.

- The size and shape of the swollen limb.
- The construction and type of compression material being used.

The size and shape of the swollen limb

The degree of compression exerted on a swollen limb is primarily governed by the circumference of the limb. This principle forms part of the Law of

Laplace which describes the relationship between applied pressure and tension in relation to the radius of a container or vessel. In lymphoedema management, this principle is relevant because limbs that have a large circumference will require a greater level of compression than limbs with a smaller circumference.

In a limb without swelling, a natural profile can be observed, with a narrow circumference at the ankle or wrist leading to a wider circumference towards the root of the limb. When compression therapy is applied to the limb, the natural profile will ensure that the greatest pressure is provided distally to encourage lymph to drain proximally.

If the limb has lost its natural profile and become misshapen because of the swelling, the circumference of the limb may vary at different points along its length and when compression is applied, care must be taken to ensure that the point of greatest pressure remains distally so that lymph drainage is not impeded. This can be achieved by ensuring that the correct choice of compression therapy is made.

The construction and type of compression material

The physical structure of the material that is applied to the swollen limb will influence the tension exerted on the limb and the subsequent response to treatment. Maximum effect is achieved through the use of inelastic materials which provide a semi-rigid outer casing to the swollen limb against which the muscles can work during exercise. The pressure on the limb is therefore high whilst the patient is moving but low when the patient is at rest, enabling the compression therapy to continue comfortably over long periods of time.

Compression garments

The daily use of a carefully fitted, comfortable compression garment is an essential aspect of lymphoedema management during the maintenance phase of treatment. A wide range of compression garments are available for both arms and legs in a variety of styles, sizes, colours and compression classes. Garments can be obtained in a ready-made format or made specially to fit the patient's individual needs.

Choosing the correct garment for the patient can be a difficult decision and should always be made with the patient's medical needs and personal considerations in mind. Table 9.2 highlights indications and contraindications in the use of compression garments. Garments can be difficult for some patients to apply and for others, difficulties may arise with the

Table 9.2   Indications and contraindications for the use of compression garments.

Indications	Rationale	Contraindications
The skin is intact with good resilience	The application and removal of compression garments can damage fragile skin	Fragile, damaged skin
The limb is a regular shape	Misshapen limbs do not fit into regular limb-shaped garments. Damage to the skin can develop if the garment does not fit well	Misshapen limbs +/− pronounced skin folds
The limb size is suitable for a garment	Compression garments must fit well to be effective and comfortable	
The excess limb volume is mild and uncomplicated	Consider bandaging to reduce limb volume prior to using compression garments	The excess limb volume is moderate/severe and complicated by poor shape and size
The patient is able to apply and remove the garment safely	Garments must be removed at night and reapplied each morning	
The patient is motivated to follow this aspect of treatment	Control of swelling can only be achieved if the garment is worn daily	
	Tissue ischaemia can occur	Arterial insufficiency
	Lymphorrhoea can be successfully managed with compression bandages	Leakage of lymph fluid (lymphorrhoea)
	The continued use of garments can be painful. Use can be resumed once the infection has been treated	Acute inflammatory episodes

appearance of the garment. Patient compliance with the use of the garment can be greatly enhanced when patient preferences are taken into account.

How compression garments work

The main aim of compression garments is to contain the swelling so that further accumulation of lymphatic fluid in the tissues is prevented. Some reduction in swelling is also possible over time but for large, complicated limbs, this can be achieved more effectively with compression bandaging.

The use of compression garments:

- limits capillary filtration
- raises the interstitial pressure in the tissues
- promotes the movement of lymph along the superficial and deep lymphatic vessels
- enhances the muscle pump action by providing an external counterforce for active muscles
- provides support for inelastic tissues.

Differences between compression garments

Construction

Compression garments are constructed in one of two ways.

- Circular, seamless knitted garments which consist of modern synthetic fibres. These garments tend to be relatively thin in texture and more aesthetically pleasing to the patient. They are readily available from a range of manufacturers and attempt to 'normalise' the appearance of the limb during wear. These garments suit a wide range of patients, particularly if the swelling is mild and uncomplicated.
- Flat-knit garments are made from a flat piece of material brought together with a seam. The material used is thicker and less elastic than circular-knit garments. Flat-knit garments can be 'made to measure' for the individual patient if careful, accurate measurements of the swollen limb are recorded. These garments are suitable for all patients with lymphoedema but particularly those with larger limbs, some limb shape alteration and those who do not fit into circular-knit garments.

Compression class

The classified compression class of a garment refers to the degree of pressure exerted by the garment on the surface of the skin it surrounds (Asmussen & Strossenreuther 2003). The pressure is measured at the ankle where it is greatest for lower limbs and the pressure gradient then gradually reduces along the length of the limb, with the lowest pressure at the thigh.

Compression garments are required to meet strict standards in yarn specification, durability, testing methods and compression gradient. There are currently three different standards (Clark & Krimmel 2006):

- British Standard 6612:1985
- French Standard ASQUAL
- German Standard RAL GZ 387:2000.

Each standard adopts different testing techniques to determine the degree of compression measured at the ankle, and the pressure range used to define each compression class differs between the standards. Table 9.3 illustrates the different compression classes according to the different standards and highlights the indications for the use of each compression class.

Style of garment

In order to obtain an effective garment that fits well and is comfortable for the patient, it is important to choose the correct style for the patient's particular needs. A key point is the inclusion of all swollen areas within the garment to ensure that swelling does not progress beyond the edge of the garment.

The garment should not constrict the limb at any point by being allowed to roll over at the edge or form ridges where a tourniquet effect can occur.

Once positioned on the limb, the garment should be firm and supportive along the length of the limb, but not tight and restrictive. There should not be any loose pockets of material where swelling can develop. The patient will need to be able to wear the garment for long periods of time, so comfort and acceptability are vital.

The colour of the garment and type of material are important considerations for some patients and every attempt should be made to acknowledge the patient's preference. Lower compression class garments are available in a wide range of lighter materials and colours and some manufacturers are now producing a wider range of garment colours in higher compression classes.

Measuring for compression garments

For lymphoedema to be successfully managed, any compression garments used by the patient must fit well. Ready-to-wear garments require basic circumferential measurement at set points on the limb to guide the therapist in choosing the correct size for the individual patient. Compression garment manufacturers provide their own tape measures and measurement charts to assist in the selection of a garment using the circumferential measurements obtained. The basic measurement points for arm and leg measurements are illustrated in Figures 9.1 and 9.2.

Table 9.3 Compression classes and indications for use.

Compression class	British Standard BS 6612:1985 Testing method: HATRA Pressure at the ankle	French Standard ASQUAL Testing method: IFTH Pressure at the ankle	German Standard RAL-GZ 387:2000 Testing method: HOSY Pressure at the ankle	Indications for use in lymphoedema management
Class 1: Mild compression	14–17 mm/Hg	10–15 mm/Hg	18–21 mm/Hg	• Early, mild lymphoedema • Minimal or no shape distortion • Active patients • Elderly patients • Palliative care
Class 2: Medium compression	18–24 mm/Hg	15–20 mm/Hg	22–32 mm/Hg	• Moderate/uncomplicated lymphoedema • Minimal shape distortion, profile retained • Active patients • Elderly and pressure-sensitive patients with leg lymphoedema
Class 3: Strong compression	25–35 mm/Hg	20–36 mm/Hg	34–46 mm/Hg	• Moderate lymphoedema • Larger limb with some shape distortion but good limb profile • Risk of swelling rebound following compression bandaging • Active patients • Some tissue fibrosis
Class 4: Very strong compression	Unavailable	>36 mm/Hg	>49 mm/Hg	• Swelling not contained by medium or strong compression • Usually flat-knit, custom-made garments • Younger, pressure-resistant patients

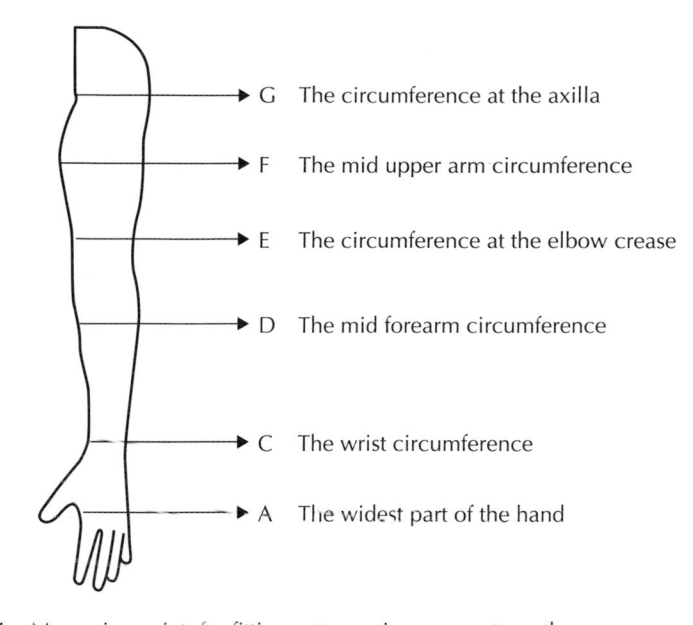

G   The circumference at the axilla

F   The mid upper arm circumference

E   The circumference at the elbow crease

D   The mid forearm circumference

C   The wrist circumference

A   The widest part of the hand

Figure 9.1   Measuring points for fitting compression garments on the arm.

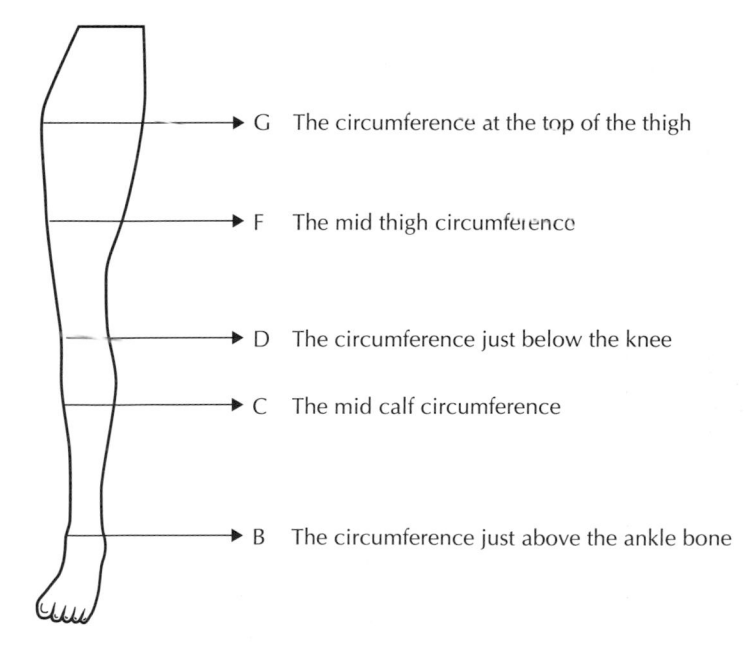

G   The circumference at the top of the thigh

F   The mid thigh circumference

D   The circumference just below the knee

C   The mid calf circumference

B   The circumference just above the ankle bone

Figure 9.2   Measuring points for fitting compression garments on the leg.

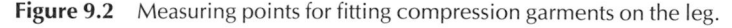

Key points

- If possible, measure the limb early rather than late in the day as further swelling may accumulate in the limb as the day progresses.
- Whilst recording measurements, the limb should be still, relaxed and resting to avoid any impact of muscle bulk.
- The tape measure should be placed evenly around the limb at the relevant measuring points to measure the circumference snugly but without applied tension.

Made-to-measure garments require a series of carefully recorded limb measurements to enable an individualised garment to be made and this measurement should be completed by a trained therapist to ensure that the final garment fits well and the possibility of expensive mistakes is avoided.

Application and removal of compression garments

It is important to educate patients in the correct way to apply and remove their compression garments. If poorly applied, the correct garment can be uncomfortable and skin damage can arise if a poor technique is used when applying or removing a garment.

The patient's ability to apply and remove their garment may be limited for a variety of reasons. Wearing an ordinary pair of household rubber gloves can protect the garment from tears and snags during application, make application much easier and ensure that the material is distributed evenly along the length of the limb. Various aids to assist in the application and removal of garments are also available commercially.

Application

- The skin should be clean and free of creams or oils which can damage the garment fibres.
- The garment should be applied early in the day when the limb is least swollen.
- With household rubber gloves on, fold the garment back on itself to wrist or ankle level and then pull on carefully in segments.
- Ensure that the material does not become bunched in one area as this can cause severe discomfort.
- Ensure that the material is evenly distributed along the length of the limb and that the garment reaches the root of the limb.
- The garment should not roll or fold over at the top and there should not be any wrinkles or tight bands of material once the garment is in place.

- The garment should never be cut or reshaped if it does not fit well and should not be folded over at the top if it is too long. It is better to consider an alternative garment if it does not fit the patient.

Removal

- Fold the garment back on itself and peel off carefully.

Wear and care of compression garments

Garments are generally worn during the day while the muscles are active and removed at night while the patient is sleeping. They should always be worn during exertive activity, sports and exercise. Wearing compression garments should not cause pain or discomfort, pins and needles or numbness in the limb. The patient should be instructed that if these symptoms do occur, the garment must be removed.

With careful use, compression garments can be used daily for a period of 4–6 months before they need replacing. The provision of two garments will ensure that one can be washed whilst the other is worn. Regular washing according to the manufacturer's recommendations with a gentle detergent will keep the garment clean and prolong its life. The garment should be dried flat, away from direct heat sources which can damage the fibres of the garment, and should not be ironed.

Compression bandages

Bandaging of any kind requires care and attention to detail to ensure the bandage is effective and comfortable for the patient. Compression bandaging in the management of lymphoedema using low-stretch bandages is a specialist technique which should not be attempted by health-care professionals without appropriate education and guidance.

The low-stretch bandages used in lymphoedema management are applied as part of a multilayer system to provide a semi-rigid encasement to the tissues. This serves as a layer of resistance against muscular pressure and the lymphatics are therefore compressed during movement.

For bandaging to be effective, the pressure exerted by the multilayer bandaging system must be evenly distributed around the circumference of the limb and graduated along the length of the limb. This can be achieved by:

- externally correcting the shape and profile of the limb with the use of foam and padding

- selecting the correct width of bandage for the circumference of the limb. A narrow bandage should be used where the circumference of the limb is small and a wider bandage where the circumference of the limb is greater
- taking care with the amount of bandage overlap to ensure it is even and graduated along the length of the limb
- applying the correct tension to the bandage during application to ensure it is even along the length of the limb.

The effectiveness of the bandaging can also be influenced by:

- the skill and technique of the therapist applying the bandages
- the nature of any physical activity carried out by the patient.

Choosing patients for compression bandaging

The decision to undertake a course of multilayer compression bandaging over a short, specified period of time should be made with careful consideration of the patient's physical and psychological ability to undertake the treatment and with clearly identified aims and objectives in mind. Tables 9.4 and 9.5 outline indications and contraindications for the use of compression bandages in lymphoedema management.

Preparing the patient for a course of compression bandaging

The patient should be appropriately prepared with verbal and written information provided regarding the following.

- *Suitable clothing.* The bandages can be bulky once in place so loose-fitting, easily applied clothes are important to ensure comfort and accommodate the bandages once they are applied.
- *Footwear.* If the leg is being bandaged, it is important that suitable footwear is worn to ensure safety whilst walking.
- *Personal hygiene.* The bandages should only be removed for a short period of time before reapplication to ensure that any reaccumulation of fluid is minimised. A daily bath or shower is possible but only if the bandages can be reapplied without delay. Accessories are available to place over a bandaged limb to keep the bandages dry during a shower. It is important that the skin is cleansed, dried carefully and moisturised with an emollient each time the bandages are removed.
- *Travel arrangements.* Compression bandages may restrict the patient's ability to react quickly to situations while driving. Patients should be

Table 9.4 Indications for the use of compression bandaging.

Indications	Rationale
A limb volume greater than 20% of the opposite limb	Larger limbs can be effectively reduced using compression bandaging (Badger et al. 2000)
Misshapen limb +/– pronounced skin folds	A large or distorted limb shape will not fit into compression garments. Bandaging can reduce volume and improve shape (Todd 2000)
Fragile, leaking or damaged skin	Compression garments will cause further damage to the skin during application, wear and removal. Bandaging will allow time for the skin to heal and control any lymphorrhoea (Jenns 2000)
Fibrotic skin changes	The semi-rigid encasement of the limb by the bandages can soften solid, non-pitting areas of tissue (Woods 2004)
Advanced malignant disease	Bandaging can offer symptomatic relief to a heavy, uncomfortable limb and be adaptive to meet the patient's needs

Table 9.5 Contraindications for compression bandaging.

Contraindications	Rationale
Arterial insufficiency	Tissue ischaemia can occur
Deep vein thrombosis	Anticoagulation therapy is required before management of any related swelling can start
Acute inflammatory episodes	The limb may be painful
Poorly controlled cardiac failure	Fluid overload can occur
Physical or psychological unsuitability of the patient to undertake the treatment	The patient needs to be compliant with treatment and able to cope with the physical bulk that results from the bandages

advised to seek advice from their insurance company if they wish to use their car during a course of compression bandaging and to consider other methods of travel if at all possible.

- *Work, family and social activities.* It is important that the patient leads as normal a life as possible whilst the bandages are in place but consideration must be given to the patient's personal circumstances and whether adjustments are required throughout the course of bandaging. In some situations, additional help may be required at home.

Supporting the patient during a course of compression bandaging

The bandages should feel comfortable at all times and not cause pain or discomfort in the limb or tingling and numbness in the digits. If discomfort of any type occurs, the patient should be instructed to first remove the top layer of bandages to see if the discomfort improves. Further layers must be removed if the discomfort persists. It is important that the patient understands that it is preferable for the bandages to be removed if there is any discomfort, rather than leaving them in place, as this will ensure their comfort and prevent the progression of any problematic factors.

Muscular activity enhances the effectiveness of compression bandages and the patient should be encouraged to be as active as possible throughout their treatment. If this is not possible, exercises to put the limb through a full range of movement or passive limb exercises should be completed daily in order to encourage a similar effect.

The following case scenarios illustrate how the different types of compression therapy can be used in the management of lymphoedema and highlight how treatment strategies may need to change.

Case Scenario 1

Peter is a 78-year-old retired army officer who lives alone. One year ago he developed a deep vein thrombosis (DVT) in his left leg and after a period of hospitalisation for anticoagulation therapy, he noticed that his left calf was swollen. He was advised that a swollen leg can develop and persist after a DVT and was fitted with a below-knee compression stocking to wear every day to help reduce the swelling and minimise the potential problem of post-thrombotic syndrome.

At a routine hospital follow-up appointment, Peter expresses concern about the stocking. He has been wearing it every day despite finding it difficult to get on but his knee has now become very swollen. This makes it difficult for him to walk.

As Peter's leg is examined, it is noticed that the stocking has been turned over at the top because it is too long. His knee is very swollen and there is still some swelling in the ankle. Peter feels that the swelling in his calf is better and wants to stop wearing the stocking.

Consider Peter's history and reflect upon his use of the compression stocking.

- Why is Peter wearing a compression stocking and is it still required?
- Why has Peter's knee become swollen?
- What advice does Peter need regarding the application of his stocking?

Following his DVT, Peter has a risk of developing post-thrombotic syndrome, a severe form of chronic venous insufficiency. This can lead to a high venous pressure in the superficial veins and cause oedema in the lower leg. Pigmentation of the skin can also occur as the products from red blood cells break down in the tissues. Post-thrombotic syndrome can develop up to five years after the acute episode of thrombosis and be painful with prolonged swelling and skin discolouration.

Compression stockings counterbalance the effects of venous hypertension which results from persistent venous obstruction and valve damage after a DVT (Prandoni et al. 2004). They also assist the muscle pump and wearing compression stockings for an initial period of six months after a diagnosis of DVT has been recommended by Brandjes et al. (1997).

Peter remains at risk of post-thrombotic syndrome due to the persistent oedema observed in his ankle, and should be advised to continue wearing compression stockings. However, the oedema should be investigated to clarify its cause and exclude other possible medical reasons. The type and style of his compression garment also require review.

All areas that are swollen should be encased within the garment to prevent the swelling progressing beyond the edge of the garment. Peter's initial swelling was focused in the calf and it is not known whether the knee was also involved at this time. However, his stocking is too long, requiring him to turn it over at the top, and the resulting tourniquet effect developing at the knee has lead to an exacerbation of the swelling.

Peter now needs a full-length compression stocking extending from the foot to the thigh. This will influence the remaining ankle oedema and the oedema in the knee. The garment chosen should be carefully fitted to ensure it is the correct compression class, size and style. Regular follow-up appointments should be made so that use of the garment can be reassessed to ensure it remains appropriate in fit until the oedema has resolved.

Peter should be advised regarding the application, removal and care of his compression stocking. Application can be aided by the use of household rubber gloves which provide a grip on the garment. By easing the stocking up his leg in segments, he is less likely to overstretch it and once fitted, the garment should feel comfortable and not be turned over on itself at any point.

Case Scenario 2

Elaine is 69 years of age and has lymphoedema in her right arm which developed several years ago following treatment for breast cancer. The swelling has been well controlled with the use of a compression sleeve which she wears daily. She lives with her husband Jim who is undergoing treatment for prostate cancer.

On their way to the hospital at the beginning of Jim's treatment, Elaine fell on an icy pavement and broke her right arm. The arm was set in plaster for four weeks and once it was removed, Elaine was advised to start wearing her compression sleeve again. Unfortunately, it no longer fitted. The arm had become more swollen and she found her sleeve too difficult to apply. By now Jim had finished his treatment and they had a holiday booked in Spain that they had been looking forward to. Elaine made an appointment to attend the lymphoedema clinic on her return from holiday.

At her appointment, her arm was found to be very swollen and mis-shapen with swelling noted in the fingers and hand. Elaine was distressed because the swelling was influencing her ability to complete her daily activities and affecting her choice of clothes because she could not get her arm into some of her sleeves. She wondered if the swelling would ever return to the controlled level it was at before she broke her arm.

Consider Elaine's history and reflect upon the history of her lymphoedema.

- Why do you think her swelling has increased?
- What strategies of lymphoedema management might she now require?
- What advice would you give Elaine?

Elaine's lymphoedema will have increased for the following reasons.

- Her arm was immobilised in a plaster and may have altered in shape as a result of the break which has been re-set.
- Although movement has now recommenced, Elaine has not been able to wear her compression sleeve for several weeks and has therefore lost control of her swelling.

It is likely that Elaine will require a course of multilayer compression band-aging to reduce the swelling and return her arm to a normal limb shape so that a new compression garment can be fitted. If she tries to wear a compression garment whilst her arm is misshapen it is possible that the swelling will become more complex. A badly fitting garment will also threaten skin integrity.

Elaine should be advised that a compression garment is not appropri-ate for her at present. If she is unable to undertake a course of multilayer

compression bandaging, a made-to-measure garment would be an alternative. In the meantime, she should ensure that she looks after her skin
by moisturising it daily as it will have become drier than normal whilst
her arm is more swollen. She should also ensure that she exercises her
arm gently to promote the return of a full range of movement and avoid
undergoing strenuous activities with the arm as these can increase lymph
production and worsen the swelling.

Conclusion

Compression therapy is an important aspect of lymphoedema management
which many patients need to undertake in order to control their swelling.
It is important that health-care professionals in all settings have an understanding of the role of compression therapy and can advise patients if
concerns about compression therapy are raised. Sources of further advice
and information should be identified in order to support patients during
this aspect of treatment.

Compression garments have an important role in the management
of lymphoedema during the maintenance phase of treatment. However,
success with their use is dependent upon the correct choice of garment
following careful consideration of the patient's needs and attention to
measuring. It is important that compression garments are perceived by
the patient as a positive aspect of treatment and that their daily wear is comfortable and, above all, acceptable. Garments should not cause distress
or influence quality of life.

Used as part of an intensive phase of management, compression bandages require greater commitment from the patient. Knowledge of the
principles underlying this specialist skill is essential and the primary role of
health-care professionals is to support their patient during this phase of
management.

References

Asmussen P. and Strossenreuther R. (2003) Compression therapy. In: M. Foldi,
    E. Foldi and S. Kubik (eds) *Textbook of Lymphology for Physicians and Lymphoedema
    Therapists*. Urban and Fischer, Germany, pp. 527–88.
Badger C.M.A., Peacock J.L. and Mortimer P.S. (2000) A randomized, controlled,
    parallel-group clinical trial comparing multi-layer bandaging followed by hosiery
    versus hosiery alone in the treatment of patients with lymphoedema of the limb.
    Cancer, **88**(12): 2832–7.
Boris M., Weindorf S., Lasinski B. and Boris G. (1994) Lymphoedema reduction by
    non-invasive complex lymphoedema therapy. *Oncology*, **8**(9): 95–106.

Brandjes D., Heijboer H. and Buller H. (1997) Randomised trial of the effect of compression stockings in patients with symptomatic proximal vein thrombosis. *Lancet*, **349**(9054): 759–62.

Callum M., Ruckley C., Dale J. and Harper D. (1997) Hazards of compression treatment of the leg: an estimate from Scottish surgeons. *British Medical Journal* (clinical research edition), **295**(6610): 1382.

Clark M. and Krimmel G. (2006) *Lymphoedema and the Construction and Classification of Hosiery. Compression Hosiery in Lymphoedema.* Medical Education Partnership, London, pp. 2–4.

Foldi E. (1985) Conservative treatment of lymphoedema. *Angiology*, **36**(3): 171–80.

Jenns K. (2000) Management strategies. In: R. Twycross, K. Jenns and J. Todd (eds) *Lymphoedema*. Radcliffe Medical Press, Oxford, pp. 97–117.

Mason M. (1993) The treatment of lymphoedema by complex physical therapy. Australian Physiotherapy, **39**(1): 41–6.

Partch H. (2003) *Understanding the Pathophysiological Effects of Compression. European Wound Management Association Position Statement: Understanding Compression Therapy.* Medical Education Partnership, London, pp. 2–4.

Prandoni P., Lensing A., Prins H. et al. (2004) Below-knee elastic compression stockings to prevent post-thrombotic syndrome. *Annals of Internal Medicine*, **141**(4): 249–56.

Todd J. (2000) Containment in the management of lymphoedema. In: R. Twycross, K. Jenns and J. Todd (eds) *Lymphoedema*. Radcliffe Medical Press, Oxford, pp. 165–202.

Woods M. (2004) External compression and support in the management of lymphoedema. In: L. Dougherty and S. Lister (eds) *The Royal Marsden Hospital Manual of Clinical Nursing Procedures*, 6th edn. Blackwell Publishing, Oxford, pp. 348–61.

10 Additional Treatments Used in the Management of Lymphoedema

Introduction

The standard management of lymphoedema follows a model of care involving a blend of the four aspects of treatment outlined in this book.

- Skin care – to promote skin integrity and minimise the risk of infection (Chapter 6).
- Exercise – to promote joint mobility and lymph drainage (Chapter 7).
- Simple/manual lymph drainage – to promote lymph drainage (Chapter 8).
- Compression – to reduce and maintain the size of the limb (Chapter 9).

Following a thorough assessment of the patient, decisions regarding the choice and timing of treatments should always be made with the patient and include consideration of the patient's ability and acceptance of the treatment proposed. Regular evaluation of progress is essential to ensure that the treatment being followed remains appropriate and manageable.

A variety of additional treatments have been reported in the management of lymphoedema and can be used in conjunction with standard management or where standard management fails. The availability of these treatments is variable and many require further evaluation of their use in lymphoedema management. However, it is important that health-care professionals have some knowledge of additional treatments in order to discuss with patients their appropriateness for the individual.

The aim of this chapter is to highlight some of the additional treatments used in the management of lymphoedema and to present the rationale behind their use.

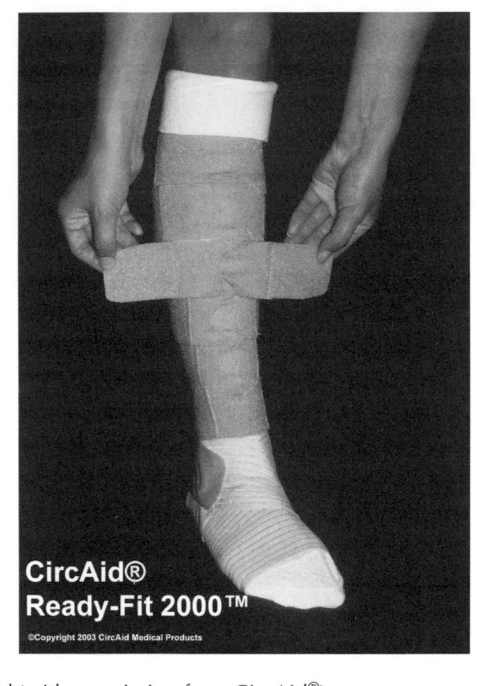

CircAid®
Ready-Fit 2000™
©Copyright 2003 CircAid Medical Products

Figure 10.1   CircAid (with permission from CircAid®).

Learning objectives

At the end of this chapter the reader will be able to:

- demonstrate knowledge of alternative and additional types of treatment useful in the management of lymphoedema
- show awareness of known indications and contraindications in the use of these treatments
- show an understanding of the role of alternative and additional types of treatment for lymphoedema when current strategies of treatment are being followed.

CircAid

The CircAid illustrated in Figure 10.1 is an inelastic garment consisting of interlocking adjustable Velcro straps that can be worn over a compression garment to provide a greater level of compression to the limb. The straps can be easily adjusted for changes in limb size or comfort when the patient is active. Because the garment is inelastic it provides sustained pressure along the length of the limb with increased compression during activity (high working pressure) and reduced compression during rest (low resting pressure).

A study by Spence & Cahall (1996) demonstrated that in a small group of patients, the inelastic CircAid achieved better maintenance of limb size than compression stockings.

Drug treatment

Lymphoedema cannot be treated with drugs alone but occasionally drugs are used in conjunction with standard management of the swelling. There are two groups of drugs which have been used:

- diuretics
- benzopyrones.

Diuretics

The administration of diuretics results in an increased excretion of water from the body. Diuretics are often incorrectly prescribed as an initial treatment for lymphoedema in the belief that a reduction in blood volume will reduce capillary filtration and lymph formation (Mortimer & O'Donnell 2003). Where oedema of mixed origin is present, diuretics may be useful but in the management of lymphoedema they have no value.

Benzopyrones

Benzopyrones are a group of naturally occurring substances, some of which have been found to be beneficial in the treatment of high-protein oedemas (Casley-Smith & Casley-Smith 1986). In the management of lymphoedema, studies involving benzopyrones have focused primarily on one group – the coumerols. Trials have produced conflicting results, however, and concerns have been raised regarding the side effect of hepatotoxicity in some patients (Loprinzi et al. 1999).

Hyperbaric oxygen

The use of high-pressure oxygen therapy is widely discussed in the literature to promote bone healing when necrosis occurs following radiotherapy and in the treatment of some orthopaedic injuries and chronic wounds.

A study exploring the use of hyperbaric oxygen in patients with brachial plexopathy following breast cancer treatment observed an unexpected finding that some patients with chronic arm lymphoedema noted a persistent improvement in their arm volume following the hyperbaric oxygen therapy (Pritchard et al. 2001). A subsequent study of the use of hyperbaric oxygen therapy in women with breast cancer-related lymphoedema (Gothard et al. 2004) observed a reduction in arm volume and a softening of the tissues of the swollen arm. These findings were limited by the absence of a control group and a further randomised controlled trial is now in progress to explore this finding further.

The aim of the study is to test the efficacy of hyperbaric oxygen therapy in reducing the development of arm lymphoedema following radiotherapy for early breast cancer. Participants randomised to hyperbaric oxygen therapy enter the hyperbaric oxygen chamber five days a week for six weeks. The chamber is pressurised and 100% oxygen is breathed for a total period of 90 minutes with a five-minute break every 30 minutes. The control group receive standard management of their lymphoedema throughout the study period. The study will help to determine whether hyperbaric oxygen offers a new approach to the management of lymphoedema.

Kinesiotaping

A relatively new concept in lymphoedema management is the use of tape, applied in a specific way to the skin in an area where lymphoedema is present. With a history of use in sports injuries (Kase et al. 2003), kinesiotape has an elastic quality which is thought to allow free physical movement whilst it is in place. Stretching of the tape during body movement is thought to encourage the skin to be lifted, taking pressure off intestinal fluid in the area of application to allow drainage of lymph fluid (Kase et al. 2003).

In the management of lymphoedema, correct positioning of the tape is considered important to facilitate drainage of lymph and channel it in the correct direction (Kase et al. 2003). Application of the tape requires knowledge of lymph drainage routes and the correct application technique for the area being treated. The tape is cut into a fan shape and applied to stretched skin to promote the development of small convolutions in the tape enabling the skin to be lifted during movement. Figure 10.2 illustrates kinesiotape applied to the skin. The fan shape is anchored close to normal draining lymph nodes and spread out over the adjacent swollen area so that lymph is drawn towards the lymph nodes to drain away.

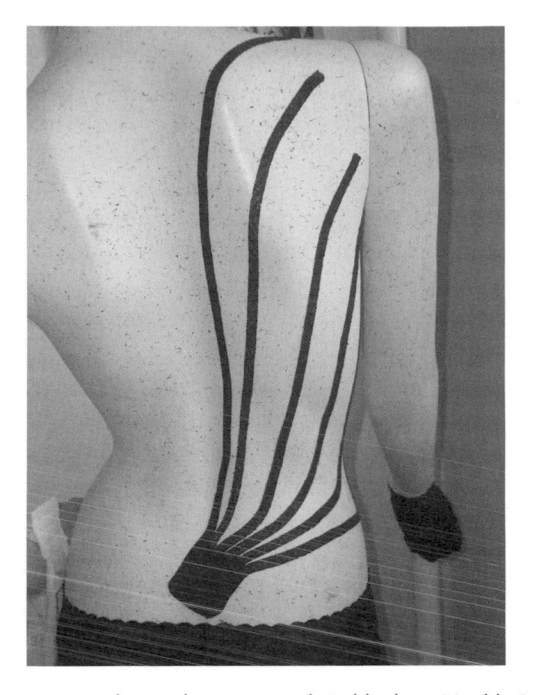

Figure 10.2   Kinesiotape on the trunk (courtesy of Haddenham Health Care).

Considerations in the use of kinesiotaping

- Practitioners should be trained in the use of the tape prior to its use with patients who have lymphoedema.
- Skin irritation may occur in hypersensitive patients or if the tape is overstretched.
- The skin should be free of oil, sweat and creams prior to application of the tape to ensure it adheres to the skin.
- The tape should not be used on skin that is broken or where infection is present.
- The tape can be left in place for several days and removed by peeling it off gently in the direction of the hair growth to prevent trauma to the skin.
- Kinesiotape should not be considered as the only treatment necessary for the management of lymphoedema but rather as an addition to existing aspects of treatment.

Low-level laser therapy

Low-level laser therapy is painless and non-invasive (Twycross 2000). This type of treatment is used to assist the healing of sports injuries and provide relief from acute and chronic pain.

In lymphoedema management, low-level laser therapy is often administered in conjunction with manual lymph drainage to improve its effectiveness. Piller & Thelander (1998) used low-level laser therapy to treat lymphoedema of the arm in ten women following breast cancer treatment. The improvements noted included a softening of the tissues and a reduction in limb volume which was sustained for 36 months.

A more recent double-blind controlled trial of low-level laser therapy in postmastectomy lymphoedema by Kaviani et al. (2006) concluded that although a reduction in limb volume was observed following laser therapy, further studies are required to more accurately determine the clinical response.

Pneumatic compression pumps

This approach to the management of lymphoedema was used for many years, but its popularity declined as the benefits of an alternative conservative approach, aimed at rehabilitating and empowering the patient using physical therapies, became evident.

Pneumatic compression therapy uses compressed air, delivered via a machine, to squeeze the swollen limb. It requires an electric pump to deliver the required pressure to the limb whilst it is fully encased in a cuff which inflates and then deflates several times with the aim of squeezing the excess fluid away from the limb. Early pumps were of a single-chamber design which inflated the cuff along the whole length of the limb at the same time and then deflated again. Later models adopted a multi-chamber design with a cuff consisting of several compartments which inflate, compress and then deflate in sequence.

Studies of the use of pneumatic compression pumps do not determine the desired type of pump, appropriate pumping time or effective pressure to be used. Dini et al. (1998), in a randomised study of postmastectomy patients with lymphoedema, demonstrated that pneumatic compression pumps had a limited clinical role in the management of lymphoedema. Also, concern over their use has been expressed by Segers et al. (2002) who found a discrepancy between pressures measured inside the cuff chambers and those indicated by the device controller. Casley-Smith & Casley-Smith (1996) suggest that fragile, superficial lymphatic vessels are easily damaged by the effect of pumps, particularly when pressures exceed 60 mmHg, and that this impedes lymph drainage. In addition, the region above the edge of the cuff can become overloaded with displaced lymph fluid as the lymph vessels in this area, which may already be damaged or deficient, struggle to drain the excess fluid. Lymphoedema can therefore become problematic in the area of the trunk adjacent to the swollen limb.

Considerations in the use of pneumatic compression pumps in lymphoedema

If a pneumatic compression pump is to be used, it is important that the following factors are considered.

- The use of pumps should always be supervised by a trained therapist to ensure safety and the use of an appropriate pressure on the swollen limb.
- Pumps should never be used as the only treatment for lymphoedema. The use of compression garments or bandages between treatments will prevent fluid reaccumulating in the overstretched tissues (Bray & Barrett 2000).
- The truncal area adjacent to the limb must be free of swelling and manual lymphatic drainage must be carried out on the area following use of the pump to promote lymph drainage and prevent congestion in the area.
- If active cancer is present in the limb or adjacent truncal area, a pump should not be used as it will be painful.
- If infection is present in the limb, a pump should not be used as it will be painful and there is a risk that the infection may spread.
- A pump should not be used if the patient has a deep vein thrombosis or arterial disease.
- Pumps are expensive and should undergo regular servicing and maintenance to ensure optimum performance.

Reid sleeve

The Reid sleeve is a large tube made of compliant elastic foam which slides over the affected limb and is then secured with adjustable Velcro straps to provide a gradient of compression to the tissues underneath. The foam tube evens out the shape of the limb so that the pressure applied by the straps can be evenly graduated along the length of the limb to encourage drainage of lymph fluid.

The Reid sleeve can be fitted to an arm or a leg and is usually worn at night. The patient can apply it easily and quickly, adjusting the straps to ensure it is comfortable. No formal studies are available on its use in the management of lymphoedema.

Surgical treatment of lymphoedema

Surgery of any kind presents a risk to the individual and complications may occur. When surgery is carried out on a limb or within an area where lymphoedema is present, there is an increased risk of infection and prolonged wound healing due to the reduction in lymph flow.

Foldi & Foldi (2003) advise that there is no absolute indication for surgery in lymphoedema management whilst Kinmouth (1982) advocates surgery in the following circumstances.

- To reduce the weight of the bulky part.
- To improve the shape of the limb, making it possible for patients with large limbs to wear normal clothes again.
- To reduce the incidence of repeated infections.
- To improve the texture of the skin.

Burnand et al. (2003) suggest that current surgical treatments for lymphoedema are unable to return the swollen limb to a near normal size without scarring and if used, should aim to produce a functional limb with the optimum cosmetic result that can be achieved. Any improvement gained from surgery will require long-term maintenance with compression hosiery.

Surgical procedures used in lymphoedema management can be divided into three areas.

- Reduction procedures
- Lymphatic bypass procedures
- Liposuction

Reduction procedures

Several surgical procedures aimed at reducing the size of a grossly swollen limb are described in the literature: Homan's reducing operation, Sistrunk's reducing operation, Charles' reducing operation and Thompson's buried dermis flap operation (Burnand et al. 2003). These procedures remove excess, oedematous, subcutaneous tissue but have been criticised for causing destruction to the still functioning lymph vessels in the limb (Foldi & Foldi 2003). Most frequently used to treat lower limb lymphoedema, the procedures have also been adapted to treat swelling in the eyelids and genitalia.

Lymphatic bypass procedures

The restoration of lymphatic function has been attempted using a variety of procedures. Obstructed lymphatic vessels have been anastomosed to vessels in the venous system in an attempt to drain the swollen limb (Gloviczki 1988) and normal healthy lymph vessels have been transplanted into areas where lymphoedema exists in order to connect poorly functioning lymph vessels with normal ones (Baumeister et al. 1991). Microsurgical techniques are required for these procedures and results appear to be more successful if patients are carefully selected and in the younger age group.

Liposuction

The removal of subcutaneous fat from a large limb by suction has been used as a method of reducing limb size when standard lymphoedema management fails (Brorson & Svensson 1998). The procedure involves several incisions along the length of the limb through which a cannula is inserted. The subcutaneous fat is sucked out through the cannula under vacuum. Liposuction does not correct lymph drainage and results are only maintained through the continued use of high compression garments. Brorson et al. (1999) reported good results with this technique in women with lymphoedema of the arm whose procedures had been carried out five years earlier.

The following case scenario highlights the use of a pneumatic pump in lymphoedema management.

Case Scenario

Daphne developed lymphoedema in her right arm 25 years ago following treatment for breast cancer. The swelling appeared slowly following her breast cancer treatment and gradually, over a few years, extended from her wrist to her armpit before the size stabilised. Her doctor, although sympathetic, was unable to offer any treatment.

After several years, Daphne's husband Jack read a magazine article which mentioned a pneumatic compression pump that could be used to remove fluid from the arm. Their doctor could see no reason why Daphne could not try the pump, so Jack purchased one from the company for Daphne and they were advised on its use.

Over the next 20 years Daphne used the compression pump every day. She set it up every morning and spent the first two hours of every day attending to her arm. Holidays were taken locally so that the pump could be taken along and easily plugged into the electrical supply and when they stayed in a hotel, Daphne always had breakfast in their room whilst she was attached to the pump. The pump never broke down or needed any maintenance and its use seemed to soften the tissues of Daphne's arm. When the cuff was removed after use of the pump, Daphne could see the improvement it had made, but she always felt disappointed that the swelling had returned by the time she went to bed. Sometimes she would use the pump again in the afternoon for a short time if she was going out for the evening. Daily use of the pump was part of everyday life for Jack and Daphne for many years.

As lymphoedema management took on a more conservative approach, Daphne was asked one day by her doctor if she ever wore a compression sleeve on her swollen arm. He referred her to a lymphoedema service for a discussion on the management of her swollen arm to see if there was anything else she could be doing.

Initially Daphne was quite reluctant to consider any other treatment for the management of her lymphoedema and could not believe that a compression sleeve would be of any additional benefit to her. She continued to use her pneumatic compression pump every morning, but started to wear a compression sleeve during the day and was surprised to notice that her swelling did not seem so bad at the end of the day. Eventually she wondered if she could manage to have a 'day off' the pump and Jack persuaded her to try.

Over the next few months Daphne used the pump less and less until she eventually decided to stop using it altogether. She did not mind wearing a compression sleeve and was delighted to see that it was controlling her swelling well.

Consider what you know of Daphne and Jack.

- What impact do you think the use of the pump had on Daphne's quality of life?

Daphne and Jack incorporated the pneumatic compression pump into their daily lives because they believed it would help to control Daphne's lymphoedema. Although this may have been the case, there are some issues that need acknowledging.

- The pump aged over time and was not serviced or checked for accuracy. As Daphne's use of the pump was not monitored she may have been receiving an inappropriate level of compression to her swollen arm.
- Daphne was linked up to a machine for a few hours each day. This influenced her ability to 'normalise' the condition of lymphoedema and incorporate the swelling into her daily life. Instead she was ruled by the machine to the point that her choice of holiday was affected.

- Daphne did not use any additional aspect of management for her lymphoedema so the perceived benefits gained by the use of the pump were gradually lost.
- Continued use of the machine over such a long period of time may mean that its benefit is overestimated by the patient.

Conclusion

A variety of treatments have been proposed in the management of lymphoedema in addition, or as an alternative, to the conservative model of management most frequently adopted. It is important that patients are able to discuss their interest in other treatments with health-care professionals who are able to advise them or direct them towards further information.

Many of the treatments discussed in this chapter require further evaluation and should not be used in isolation. Patients should therefore be encouraged to continue with management strategies which have a stronger physiological basis for their use, incorporating other treatment approaches if they wish after discussion and under the direction of a trained health-care professional.

References

Baumeister R., Frick A. and Hofmann T. (1991) Ten years experience with autogenous microsurgical lymph vessel-transplantation. *European Journal of Lymphology*, **6**: 62.

Bray T. and Barrett J. (2000) Pneumatic compression therapy. In: R. Twycross, K. Jenns and J. Todd (eds) *Lymphoedema*. Radcliffe Medical Press, Oxford, pp. 236–43.

Brorson H. and Svensson H. (1998) Liposuction combined with controlled compression therapy reduces arm lymphoedema more effectively than controlled compression therapy alone. *Plastic and Reconstructive Surgery*, **102**: 1058–67.

Brorson H., Adberg M. and Svennson H. (1999) Complete reduction of arm lymphoedema by liposuction following breast cancer – 5 year results. *Lymphology*, **33**(supplement): 250–3.

Burnand K., Gloviczki P. and Browse N. (2003) Principles of surgical treatment. In: N. Browse, K. Burnand and P. Mortimer (eds) *Diseases of the Lymphatics*. Arnold/Oxford University Press, London, pp. 179–204.

Casley-Smith J. and Casley-Smith J. (1986) High protein oedemas and the benzopyrones. In: J. Casley-Smith and J. Casley-Smith (eds) *History of the Lymphatics*. Lippincott, Sydney, pp. 2–3.

Casley-Smith J. and Casley-Smith J. (1996) The dangers of pumps in lymphoedema therapy. *Lymphology*, **29**(2)(supplement): 32–4.

Dini D., Del Mastro L., Gozza A. et al. (1998) The role of pneumatic compression in the treatment of postmastectomy lymphoedema. A randomised phase III study. *Annals of Oncology*, **9**(2): 187–90.

Foldi E. and Foldi M. (2003) Lymphostatic diseases. In: Foldi M., Foldi E. and Kubik S. (eds) *Textbook of Lymphology for Physicians and Lymphoedema Therapists*. Urban and Fischer, Germany, pp. 232–319.

Gloviczki P. (1988) Microsurgical lymphovenous anastomosis for treatment of lymphoedema: a critical review. *Journal of Vascular Surgery*, **7**(5): 647–52.

Gothard L., Stanton A., MacLaren J. et al. (2004) Non-randomised phase II trial of hyperbaric oxygen therapy in patients with chronic arm lymphoedema and tissue fibrosis after radiotherapy for early breast cancer. *Radiotherapy and Oncology*, **70**(3): 217–24.

Kase K., Wallis J. and Kase T. (2003) *Clinical Therapeutic Application of the Kinesio-taping Method*. Scrip, Tokyo.

Kaviani A., Fateh M., Nooraie R., Alinagizadeh M. and Fashtami L. (2006) Low level laser therapy in the management of post-mastectomy lymphoedema. *Lasers in Medical Science*, **21**(2): 90–4.

Kinmouth J. (1982) *The Lymphatics*, 2nd edn. Edward Arnold, London.

Loprinzi C., Kugler J. and Sloan J. (1999) Lack of effect of coumarin in women with lymphoedema after treatment for breast cancer. *New England Journal of Medicine*, **340**(5): 346–50.

Mortimer P. and O'Donnell T. (2003) Principles of medical and physical treatment. In: N. Browse, K. Burnand and P. Mortimer (eds) *Diseases of the Lymphatics*. Arnold/Oxford University Press, London, pp. 167–78.

Piller N. and Thelander A. (1998) Treatment of chronic postmastectomy lymphoedema with low level laser therapy: a 25 year follow-up. *Lymphology*, **31**(2): 74–86.

Pritchard J., Anand A. and Broome J. (2001) Double-blind randomised phase II study of hyperbaric oxygen therapy in patients with radiation-induced brachial plexopathy. *Radiotherapy and Oncology*, **58**(3): 279–86.

Segers P., Belgrado J-P., Leduc A., Leduc O. and Verdonck P. (2002) Excessive pressure in multichambered cuffs used for sequential compression therapy. *Physical Therapy*, **82**(10): 1000–8.

Spence R. and Cahall E. (1996) Inelastic versus elastic compression in chronic venous insufficiency: a comparison of limb size and venous haemodynamics. *Journal of Vascular Surgery*, **24**(5): 783–7.

Twycross R. (2000) Novel treatments: low level laser therapy. In: R. Twycross, K. Jenns and J. Todd (eds) *Lymphoedema*. Radcliffe Medical Press, Oxford, pp. 22–43.

11 Living with Lymphoedema

Introduction

Although lymphoedema cannot be cured, it can be effectively managed with appropriate non-invasive care. Living with lymphoedema can be challenging, however, and because it is a chronic condition that is likely to be life-long, some adaptation to aspects of daily life is always required if the swelling is to be controlled. This is easier for some than for others and an understanding of how people adjust to a chronic condition can help the health-care professional understand the individual's response to the condition.

With care, the quality of life experienced by patients with lymphoedema should not be compromised and this chapter will explore some of the areas that can be influenced by the development of swelling and consider ways in which the quality of life of an individual with lymphoedema can be maintained.

Learning objectives

At the end of this chapter the reader will be able to:

- describe the response to a chronic condition and relate this to the patient with lymphoedema
- discuss the impact of lymphoedema on a patient's emotions and relationships
- discuss the influence of lymphoedema on body image, physical activity and occupation
- outline some approaches required for the self-management of lymphoedema.

Lymphoedema as a chronic condition

Any chronic condition can have an impact upon an individual's life, causing a permanent alteration from what previously was viewed as 'normal'. Bleeker & Mulderij (1992) suggest that in illness the body 'loses its silence', drawing attention to the fact that all is not as it used to be.

Lymphoedema of the limbs is visible to the patient affected and frequently leads to attempts to disguise it (Williams et al. 2004). This physical alteration from a perception of normal can lead to feelings of being stigmatised (Hare 2000), particularly if negative social reactions are received. The more visible the condition, the more stigmatised the individual patient can feel and attempts to pass themselves off as 'normal' can lead to a fear of discovery and the subsequent need for explanation.

Johansson (2002) suggests that many patients with lymphoedema adopt a problem-focused way of coping with their swelling by attempting to change their environment and make life easier for themselves, perhaps by avoiding a certain task or activity. However, other patients will accept the way things are and adjust their values to reflect the situation in which they find themselves. This 'emotion-focused' way of coping supports the observation that many patients with lymphoedema do appear to cope well.

A key approach to the management of any chronic condition, including lymphoedema, is the setting of patient-focused goals which help the individual to aim for and realise their maximum potential. This approach is viewed as part of a restoration or healing and involves good communication coupled with education of the patient and their family (Jenns 2000, Mason 2000). The patient needs to maintain a sense of ownership for decisions and actions relating to the management of their lymphoedema, and achieving success in following a self-care regime necessary for the management of their lymphoedema provides the patient with the tools to face the challenges that a chronic condition can pose.

The impact of lymphoedema

Lymphoedema is a personal and unique experience for the individual and the response to its appearance is shaped by factors such as culture, upbringing and support from family and friends, in addition to knowledge and information gained about the condition. Table 11.1 illustrates how lymphoedema can affect an individual and highlights the areas that will be discussed throughout this chapter.

Table 11.1   Living with lymphoedema.

The potential impact of lymphoedema	Emotions Relationships
The potential influence of lymphoedema	Body image Physical activity Occupation
Aspects involved in adaptation to lymphoedema	Holidays and travel Foot care Healthy eating The role of the health-care professional Support groups

Emotions

The realisation that lymphoedema is a life-long condition can be difficult for the patient to accept and may result in a mixture of emotions. The depth of these feelings may vary and be influenced by the impact and influence of the swelling on the individual.

- *Anger.* It is not easy to accept that lymphoedema has developed, particularly if the 'at-risk' limb has been looked after in order to minimise the risk of its development. Anger can vary in strength and at times it can be difficult to see anything but the negative aspects of living with lymphoedema. Relaxation and calming activities can help to keep things in perspective so that positive approaches can be identified.
- *Depression.* Feelings of loss and sadness can develop as the patient with lymphoedema begins to realise that a change in their life is required in order to accommodate the impact of the swelling (Hare 2000). The symptoms of depression vary but may include disturbed sleep, lack of energy, tearfulness and loss of self-esteem. The sharing of feelings and thoughts can help and professional treatment for depression may be required if symptoms are severe.
- *Anxiety.* The threat to the physical well-being of the body experienced when lymphoedema develops can lead to the flight-or-fight response known as anxiety. Lymphoedema can cause certain situations and events to be perceived as stressful, particularly if the situation has not been experienced before, and anxiety regarding these situations can cause physical symptoms such as sweating, blushing, shaking and nausea which can be distressing for the patient concerned. Coping skills include relaxation techniques, and the development of an understanding of the circumstances that cause anxiety can be helpful.

Relationships

Self-esteem and confidence can be challenged by the development of lymphoedema and the patient affected can at times feel isolated with a condition that appears to demand so many considerations. Support and understanding from family and friends can lead to a positive approach in adaptation (Hare 2000).

- *Social relationships.* The patient with lymphoedema does not change because of the swelling and hobbies and activities previously shared with family and friends should not need to be discontinued. Some adaptation, such as reducing the time spent on a particular sport or activity, may be required to prevent the swelling getting worse and new activities should always be approached slowly over a longer period of time to ensure that the swelling does not worsen.
- *Sexual relationships.* There is no reason why sexual relationships with a partner should cease because of lymphoedema but when swelling is present in the genital area, care should be taken to ensure that trauma to the area is avoided. If difficulties develop, alternative ways of gaining pleasure may need to be explored and professional advice is sometimes required.
- *Personal relationships.* Many individuals with lymphoedema find it easy to 'get on with their life', adopting a direct, rational approach to the management of their swelling. Others find it more difficult, adopting a passive approach in an attempt to hide from the reality of the situation. The approach taken is thought to be related to personality type (Langens & Morth 2003) and finding ways to master different and difficult situations takes time, understanding and support from family and friends.

The influence of lymphoedema

The influence of lymphoedema upon an individual's quality of life depends upon the degree and severity of the swelling. For some patients, physical changes, as outlined in Table 11.2, can be experienced in the swollen limb and provide a constant reminder of the condition.

Body image

Our body image is formed in a personal and social context and is a vulnerable part of our persona. Most people experience some discontent with an aspect of their body at times; it may be their height, weight, hair colour or

Table 11.2   Physical changes in the limb and their potential influence.

Physical change	Potential influence
Swelling involving the fingers and hand	<ul><li>The wearing of jewellery, e.g. rings, watches, bracelets, becomes difficult</li><li>Difficulty in fine motor movements may occur</li></ul>
Swelling involving the feet	<ul><li>Difficulties choosing suitable footwear</li></ul>
Alteration in the shape of the limb due to the distribution of the swelling	<ul><li>Difficulties in choosing and wearing clothes</li><li>Influence on body image</li></ul>
Changes in the texture of the skin and tissues	<ul><li>Increased risk of infection</li></ul>
Alteration in sensation throughout the limb	<ul><li>Difficulty with fine finger movements</li><li>Potential damage to the skin through trauma</li></ul>
Increased heaviness of the limb	<ul><li>Difficulty with movement</li><li>Difficulty with limb function</li><li>Reduced spatial awareness</li></ul>

particular facial or body features. Our body image is influenced by culture, upbringing, fashion and the media who place increasing importance on the achievement of a perfect body, free of all physical imperfections. The visible, physical alteration from the 'normal' appearance of a limb due to lymphoedema can damage confidence in a patient's body image. The problem can be further exacerbated if compression garments are required to manage the swelling as more attention can be drawn to the area affected.

Price (1990) describes three components to body image.

- *Body reality*: the body as it is.
- *Body ideal*: the preferred look and function of the body.
- *Body presentation*: the way the body is presented to the world in order to balance body reality with body ideal.

When a patient has lymphoedema, however mild, the reality of their body can be in sharp conflict with their ideal or how they would like it to be. The patient has to be aware of activities and actions that may affect the swollen limb and acutely alert to changes that may occur in the condition of the limb. The body no longer looks and functions as it did and the patient is reminded that a change has occurred.

The public part of body image is how the body is presented to the world and usually involves appropriate fashion and cosmetics to present the body as healthy and attractive. People who do not achieve this may be treated differently and may experience a loss of self-esteem and confidence.

Adjusting to a change in body image can be easier for some than others. Neill & Barrell (1998) suggest that patients undergo a period of transition during which they move through three stages to reach a restructuring of their body reality and then finally come to terms with a new body image. If the patient is unprepared for the possibility that lymphoedema may develop as a result of their cancer treatment, the emotions of anger, depression and anxiety may influence the time taken to complete the period of transition. During this time support from health-care professionals, family and friends will be required.

Physical activity

The effect of physical activity on an individual's lymphoedema will be determined by the type of activity followed and the area of the body influenced by the swelling. Some activities can enhance drainage of the swelling and others appear to exacerbate swelling.

Although it can be difficult to determine an appropriate level of activity, there is no reason why the development of lymphoedema, or the risk of its appearance, should mean that a favourite sport or activity has to be discontinued, but any ache, pain or increased swelling in a limb will indicate that a review of the activity is required. New activities, particularly those of an exertive, strenuous nature and those involving repetitive or static movements, should be approached with caution until any effect upon the lymphoedema can be determined.

Occupation

A number of occupation-related issues may need to be considered by the individual with lymphoedema depending upon the type of occupation being followed, the site and degree of the swelling. This can cause distress if a change in occupation has to be considered, particularly if there are financial implications.

Patients with lymphoedema of the arm who were in employment were shown to have a greater degree of swelling than those who did not work (Woods 1995). This may reflect the additional demands placed upon a swollen limb when work activities are combined with the demands of a home and family life.

If difficulties are being experienced, the patient needs to discuss whether there are any adaptations to the work environment or alternative aspects to the role that can be considered. Simple changes can sometimes make a big difference and avoid the need to seek alternative employment.

Adapting to lymphoedema

With time, patients can become experts in managing their lymphoedema (Williams et al. 2004). They become able to judge the influence that particular activities of the day will have upon their swelling and make choices concerning the treatment required to maintain stability of their swelling.

Holidays and travel

Extended periods of inactivity during travel on long journeys can lead to a worsening of any swelling. Sitting for too long in a cramped position or standing for too long in one position can lead to a pooling of lymph fluid because of limited muscular activity.

It is important that patients with lymphoedema plan their travel arrangements carefully, taking regular breaks for some exercise if possible. Even simple movements of the affected limb whilst travelling can make a positive difference. If compression garments have been provided to manage the lymphoedema, these should always be worn during travel and upon arrival at the destination to ensure that any swelling that may have accumulated is encouraged to drain.

Wearing loose, comfortable clothes for travelling will minimise constriction of a swollen limb from tight clothing. Any luggage should be portable and as light as possible and it is advisable to make good use of luggage trolleys to move luggage around at airports and stations.

When preparing for a holiday, consideration should be given to whether there is likely to be any exposure to the sun and subsequent risk of sunburn. A high-factor suncream, loose cotton clothes and avoidance of the hot midday sun will protect the skin. A different climate can dry the skin, so extra moisturising is advisable with a non-perfumed emollient cream or lotion. Care will also be required to protect the skin from mosquitoes, using a good insect repellent.

Foot care

When lymphoedema involves the feet, foot hygiene and protection of the skin are essential. Swollen feet are prone to fungal infections between the toes and the skin can easily be damaged by friction from poorly fitting shoes.

- The skin should be examined daily for signs of skin or nail problems. Rough skin can be carefully removed following softening and a good foot cream will ensure that the skin remains supple. Nails should be trimmed with nail clippers and foot problems such as corns or calluses should always be treated by a chiropodist.
- Footwear should always be worn to protect the feet. Getting into the habit of wearing slippers in the home, sandals on the beach and shoes or boots in the garden will ensure that the feet are protected from injury. Carefully chosen footwear that is well fitting and supportive will maintain the shape of the foot. The presence of a smooth lining will protect the skin from rubbing. A low heel is preferable and comfortable, stylish, afford-able styles can be found on the high street or through specialist mail order companies. An 'odd size' service is available from some manufac-turers if one foot requires a larger size than the other. Footwear should be chosen during the early part of the day before the feet become swollen.
- Ill-fitting footwear will compromise safety and comfort. Shoes may slip off during wear if they are too big or cause friction of the skin if they are too small. A misshapen foot can develop from poorly fitting shoes which will then make the wearing of compression garments more difficult.
- Lymph drainage from the feet and legs can be encouraged with gentle foot exercises performed at regular intervals during the day and the use of a footstool to support the legs when sitting for long periods. Standing in one position for long periods should be avoided as this can cause pooling of lymph in the extremities.

Healthy eating

Maintaining a healthy body weight is considered important in the control of lymphoedema and maintenance of a reduced limb volume (Shaw 2004). Being overweight means that the swollen limb is heavier and this may result in joint or musculoskeletal problems. It also means that the muscle pump is less efficient due to the excess tissues in the limb and lymph drainage may be compromised.

Although there is no special diet that should be followed by patients with lymphoedema, a wide variety of foods chosen from all the food groups will assist in healthy eating patterns and provide other long-term health benefits.

The role of the health-care professional

When viewing the patient's lymphoedema from a professional angle, it is sometimes hard for the health-care professional to understand the degree of impact and influence that lymphoedema has upon the patient and their circumstances. But providing an opportunity for the patient to express their views and listening to their story can alleviate a lot of distress and help the patient move towards acceptance of their swelling and the achievement of successful management.

All health-care professionals have a role in supporting patients with lymphoedema. By becoming aware of the problems and worries that concern this group of patients, the health-care professional can encourage patients to continue a self-care approach to the management of their swelling knowing that support and advice are available when needed.

Support groups

Support groups offer the opportunity for patients to meet others with their condition in order to gain support from each other. A national patient-led organisation for patients with lymphoedema, the Lymphoedema Support Network, provides a wide range of written information and a strong support network for patients, their friends and families. The Lymphoedema Support Network has also developed strong links with health-care professionals working with lymphoedema patients through the British Lymphology Society. The details of both of these organisations can be found in the Useful Addresses section at the end of the book.

The following case scenario discusses the impact of lymphoedema upon the life of a young man.

Case Scenario

Paul is a 27-year-old student attending a further education college where he is studying to be a plumber. When he was 24 his girlfriend persuaded him to have a mole removed from his left ankle because she noticed it was dark and had started to bleed while they were on holiday. Paul was shocked to find that the mole was a malignant melanoma. A year later he underwent a groin dissection after noticing an enlarged lymph node which he was told was metastatic disease from his melanoma. Immediately after his surgery, Paul noticed that his leg was beginning to swell but he did not pay much attention to it. He started his course in plumbing and after a while began to get annoyed with the swelling because it affected his left foot and leg and made his trainers and shoes feel uncomfortable. He also noticed that his jeans were tight on that leg and found that he needed trouser styles that had baggy legs to accommodate his larger leg.

His training as a plumber involves long periods of time cramped in small areas in one position and this makes his knee hurt and leg ache at the end of the day. When he is in college, he finds sitting listening to lectures difficult, unless he is lucky enough to find a seat with plenty of leg room.

Consider Paul's brief history and reflect upon the impact that the lymphoedema in his leg may have upon him. Consider his age and occupation, social and psychological factors.

- What may be the long-term implications of living with lymphoedema for Paul?
- What support and advice do you think he needs?

Paul is a young man upon whom the impact of lymphoedema may be considerable. It is unlikely that his proposed occupation as a plumber will need to be reviewed, but aspects of his role will require consideration. He will need to ensure that he is able to move around whilst working and not remain in cramped positions for long periods of time. By incorporating some regular physical activity such as swimming, walking or an alternative sport into his lifestyle, lymph drainage will be promoted.

In order to control the lymphoedema, Paul will need to consider compression therapy as part of his life for the foreseeable future. Depending upon the shape of his leg, this may be in the form of a garment or a planned short course of compression bandaging followed by the daily wearing of a compression garment. The wearing of a compression garment may have an impact upon Paul's body image; as a young man, he may perceive compression stockings as a female item of clothing that is not acceptable to his male image. He may also worry about how his friends will react if they find out he is wearing a stocking and how it will affect his relationship with his girlfriend. It may be more acceptable to him to wear the garment for short periods of time only at first, increasing the occasions and time the garment is worn as he feels able. In this way Paul will gain confidence in the use of the garment and its effect upon his swelling.

It is important that personal hygiene is addressed to ensure that Paul is aware of the importance of foot care and the maintenance of skin integrity. If the health-care professional can initiate discussions in a careful manner, Paul will be encouraged to take responsibility for looking after his skin.

It is possible that the impact of a long-term condition will influence Paul's emotions. He may react with anger and refuse to follow the advice he receives. He will require support from family and friends, with his girlfriend occupying an important role in his adaptation to the condition. He will also require regular contact with a health-care professional with knowledge of lymphoedema management to ensure that any problems are identified early and that compression garments are reviewed and replaced regularly.

Conclusion

By playing a central role in the management of their condition and working in partnership with health-care professionals, patients with lymphoedema can become active participants in the management of their swelling. Recognising the individuality of each patient, their reaction to the development of lymphoedema and the impact it has upon the different roles they have in their lives means that the health-care professional can provide appropriate, well-timed advice and information. This in turn will significantly improve the patient's experience of the treatment process and encourage them to achieve success in managing the condition in their daily lives.

References

Bleeker H. and Mulderij K. (1992) The experience of motor disability. *Phenomenology and Pedagogy*, **4**(2): 44–53.

Hare M. (2000) The lived experience of breast cancer-related lymphoedema. *Nursing Standard*, **15**(7): 35–9.

Jenns K. (2000) Management strategies. In: R. Twycross, K. Jenns and J. Todd (eds) *Lymphoedema*. Radcliffe Medical Press, Oxford, pp. 97–117.

Johansson K. (2002) Lymphoedema and breast cancer: a physiotherapeutic approach. PhD thesis, Department of Physical Therapy, Lund University, Sweden.

Langens T. and Morth S. (2003) Repressive coping and the use of passive and active coping strategies. *Patientality and Individual Differences*, **35**(2): 461–73.

Mason W. (2000) Exploring rehabilitation within lymphoedema management. *International Journal of Palliative Nursing*, **6**(6): 265–73.

Neill J. and Barrell L. (1998) Transition theory and its relevance to patients with chronic wounds. *Rehabilitation Nursing*, **23**(6): 295–9.

Price B. (1990) A model for body-image care. *Journal of Advanced Nursing*, **15**(5): 585–93.

Shaw C. (2004) *Dietary Interventions*. Annual Research Report: The Royal Marsden NHS Foundation Trust and Institute of Cancer Research, London, pp. 58–61.

Williams A., Moffatt C. and Franks P. (2004) A phenomenological study of the lived experiences of people with lymphoedema. *International Journal of Palliative Nursing*, **10**(6): 279–86.

Woods M. (1995) Sociological and psychological implications of lymphoedema. *International Journal of Palliative Nursing*, **1**(1): 17–20.

12 Complications of Lymphoedema

Introduction

Occasionally lymphoedema presents with interrelated problems which may be reported by the patient or clinically observed by the health-care professional during an assessment of the swollen area or general consultation with the patient. Although these situations should be managed by specialists with appropriate knowledge and skills, it is important that health-care professionals are able to recognise when lymphoedema has become complicated so that an appropriate referral for further advice and management can be made.

Learning objectives

At the end of this chapter the reader will be able to:

- outline some of the complications that can occur when lymphoedema develops
- recognise when lymphoedema may be complicated and know when to refer to a specialist for further advice
- describe the reasons why a swollen limb may become impaired in function
- identify the causes of lymphorrhoea and outline the management of the condition
- describe the characteristics of pain in a swollen limb
- outline the venous complications that may influence management of lymphoedema.

Chronic lymphoedema

Without appropriate management of the limb, lymphoedema can become progressive and advanced. The International Society of Lymphology (2000) describes the characteristics of Stage 3 lymphoedema as follows.

- Severe skin changes.
- The skin loses elasticity and develops skin folds.
- The risk of infection increases and the limb volume difference is greater than 40%.

Foldi & Foldi (2003) consider lymphoedema to be spontaneously irreversible at this stage requiring complex, specialist therapy to gain control of the swelling and achieve maximum improvement in the size, shape and condition of the limb. Figure 12.1 illustrates advanced lymphoedema of an arm which developed following breast cancer treatment and was treated with compression bandaging and manual lymphatic drainage. After several weeks, compression garments could be fitted to maintain control of the improvement gained.

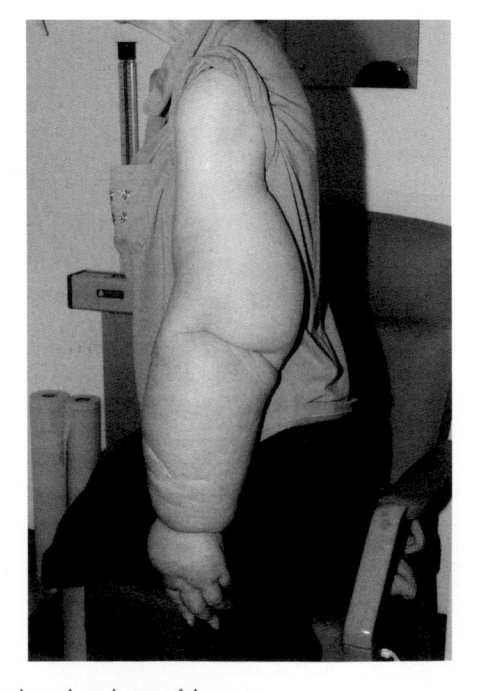

Figure 12.1   Chronic lymphoedema of the arm.

Compression therapy complications

Compression therapy is an important aspect of the management of lymphoedema and a patient's suitability for this aspect of management should be established following a full assessment, as outlined in Chapter 5.

Complications can occur if the principles of compression therapy, detailed in Chapter 9, are not followed or if the effect of the compression therapy is not regularly evaluated, with subsequent adjustments made if necessary.

The following complications can be caused by poor technique and poor evaluation:

- skin breakdown due to pressure areas developing following poor application of the garment/bandages
- a tourniquet effect on the limb and reduced blood supply to the limb due to a poorly fitted garment/poorly applied bandages
- pain in the limb due to the garment/bandages being too tight
- inappropriate compression provided by the garment/bandages causing discomfort and potential ischaemia of the limb.

Complications arising as a result of compression therapy can be difficult to manage, in very severe cases can lead to the loss of a limb and are avoidable.

Impaired function

The movement and function of a limb can become impeded when lymphoedema is present. The swelling can make the limb heavy and cumbersom, resulting in a reduction in the normal range of movement. Swelling affecting the hand and fingers causes a weakening of grip and difficulties with, or even loss of, fine finger movements. Reduced dexterity will impede everyday activities and spatial awareness may be affected as movement of a heavy, swollen limb becomes difficult to control. The function and mobility of a swollen limb can be improved with appropriate treatment of the lymphoedema (Sitzia & Sobrido 1997).

Musculoskeletal effects

Over time, a heavy limb will have an impact upon associated joints and muscles. Patients with arm lymphoedema may experience shoulder and neck discomfort whilst patients with leg oedema may experience hip and back problems as the heavy limb results in an unequal balance of body weight.

Brachial plexopathy

The area treated with radiation therapy for breast cancer treatment may include the brachial plexus nerve and in some cases this treatment may result in radiation-induced fibrosis. Symptoms can take several years to appear and gradually affect the sensory and motor functions of the arm. The patient will complain of progressive loss of sensation in the fingers and hand which gradually leads to weakness and loss of function. Brachial plexopathy can be painful and advice concerning management of the associated neuropathic pain will be required. The condition is irreversible and can cause a significant impact upon quality of life.

In metastatic disease the brachial nerve may be infiltrated with tumour in the supraclavicular region. Symptoms reported by the patient include pain associated with a loss of function. Appropriate oncological management can result in regression of the disease and an improvement in the symptoms.

Lymphorrhoea

Identification

Lymphorrhoea is a complication of oedema in which lymph weeps in beads of fluid through the surface of the skin (Linnett 2000). The fluid is straw coloured with a slight odour and stickiness. Several areas of the skin may leak at the same time, forming steady trickles of fluid, the volume of which can be significant over a period of time. Lymphorrhoea in a leg is illustrated in Figure 12.2.

Causes

Lymphorrhoea can develop in the following situations:

- following trauma to oedematous skin
- when oedematous skin becomes scaly and hypertrophic
- following the rapid development of oedema when the skin is thin and fragile; the increased pressure causes the skin to leak
- following the herniation of lymphatic vessels through the surface of the skin (acquired lymphangiomata).

Problems associated with lymphorrhoea

If left untreated, lymphorrhoea can continue for several days, leaking through dressings and clothes and putting the surrounding skin at risk of

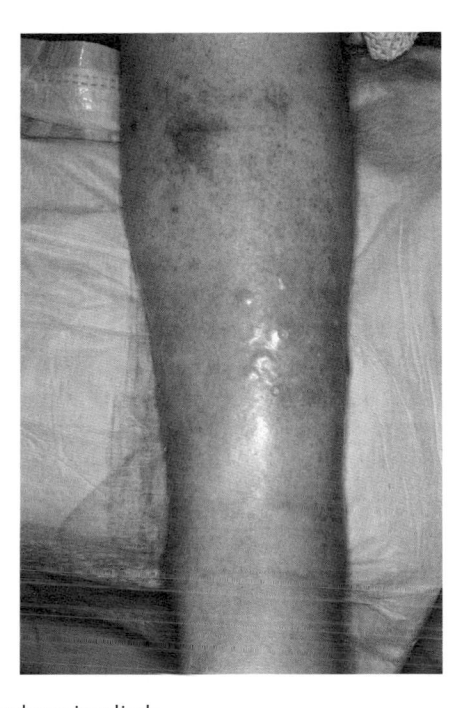

Figure 12.2   Lymphorrhoea in a limb.

maceration through the presence of continued moisture. The limb feels cold and uncomfortable to the patient and the continued leaking creates problems with clothes, shoes and bedding.

There is a significant risk of infection through broken, traumatised skin and fragile skin can be further traumatised by the use of dressings and tape over the leaking areas.

Managing lymphorrhoea

The immediate aims are to:

- stop the leakage of fluid and prevent skin maceration
- improve patient comfort
- minimise the risk of infection
- prevent further trauma to the skin.

It is not appropriate to allow the leakage to continue and health-care professionals can initiate early management, prior to specialist intervention, in order to avoid further complications. This is highlighted in Table 12.1.

Ling et al. (1997), in a survey of palliative care units, highlighted a limited evidence base for the management of lymphorrhoea. The choice of dressings

Table 12.1   The early management of lymphorrhoea.

Action	Rationale
Cleanse the skin with warm soapy water	To remove the residue of lymph fluid from the skin
Dry the skin thoroughly	To prevent maceration of the skin
Moisturise the skin well with an emollient	To improve skin integrity
Apply a sterile, non-adherent dressing to absorb the fluid and secure with a retention bandage	Tape should not be used as it will traumatise the skin
Slightly elevate the area of leakage if possible. A limb should be positioned at heart level	To reduce hydrostatic pressure
Renew dressings if they become wet	To prevent maceration of the skin and promote patient comfort
Seek advice from a specialist experienced in the use of compression bandages	To initiate care of the limb to stop the leakage of lymph fluid

Table 12.2   Managing lymphorrhoea in a limb.

- Cleanse and moisturise the skin.
- Apply non-adherent dressings to all areas of leakage and secure in place with light retention bandages. Do not use tape.
- Apply a cotton Tubifast bandage to the skin to provide protection from any friction as the compression bandages are applied.
- Apply padding over the Tubifast to even out the shape of the limb.
- Compression bandages are then applied to the length of the limb in a firm, supportive manner to provide pressure on the tissues.
- The bandages can be left in place for 24–48 hours unless they become moist and require renewal to prevent skin maceration.

varied and the use of bandages was considered problematic when ana-tomical considerations had to be made. More recent guidance (Maclaren 2001, Williams 2004, Woods 2004) has suggested that lymphorrhoea can be successfully managed with an adapted short course of low-stretch com-pression bandages applied in layers to the affected limb.

The management of lymphorrhoea is illustrated in Table 12.2. The bandages can be left in place for 24–48 hours and then carefully removed. If fluid leaks while the bandages are in place, the dressings and bandages should be replaced to prevent the skin from remaining moist and becom-ing macerated. Once the lymphorrhoea has stopped, skin care should be

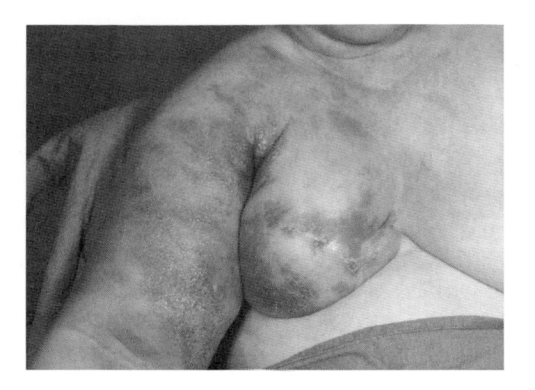

Figure 12.3   Metastatic malignant disease and arm lymphoedema.

continued to maintain skin integrity. Compression garments should be avoided until the fragile skin has improved and skin integrity has been achieved.

Malignant disease

Any patient with a history of malignancy is at risk of metastatic tumour obstruction within lymph node areas. This can lead to a sudden increase in swelling, altered sensations within a limb, pain within the limb or gradual loss of function and should always be medically investigated. Figure 12.3 illustrates the effect of metastatic malignant disease in a patient with breast cancer-related lymphoedema.

New malignancies can also occur within a swollen limb and although rarely observed, a relationship has been demonstrated between chronic lymphoedema of a limb and the development of lymphangiosarcoma (Mulvenna et al. 1995).

Lymphangiosarcoma

This rare malignant disease is aggressive and carries a poor prognosis. The diagnosis is made on skin biopsy and the clinical features include:

- a solitary purple/red focus in the skin giving the appearance of a bruise; it may be slightly raised and nodular
- single or multiple haemorrhagic nodules on the oedematous limb
- satellite tumours which develop locally on the limb and may ulcerate as they grow
- distant metastatic spread is usually pulmonary or to the chest wall.

The tumour is not responsive to chemotherapy or radiotherapy so amputation of the limb may need to be considered if the disease remains localised.

Pain

The experience of pain associated with lymphoedema in a limb should always be investigated in order to establish its cause. If the pain is of sudden onset, complications such as thrombosis or active disease will need to be considered.

Descriptions of pain vary and an assessment of the patient's pain should include the following.

- The location of the pain, using diagrams if necessary.
- The duration of the pain: details regarding its onset and whether it is acute, chronic or recurrent.
- The quality of the pain, using descriptors such as burning, searing, throbbing.
- The intensity of the pain: the worst it gets, the best it gets.
- Exacerbating factors: what makes it worse, what makes it better.
- The effect of the pain upon the patient.

A study by Carroll & Rose (1992) found that the ten words chosen from the McGill Pain Questionnaire (Melzack 1975) most frequently used to describe pain associated with lymphoedema of the arm were: *'tiring, tight, throbbing, heavy, nagging, aching, shooting, tingling, hot and annoying'*.

Pain does not occur in all patients with lymphoedema. Badger et al. (1988) reported that 43% of patients did not experience any pain but when pain does occur, it is most frequently associated with stretching of the tissues due to the oedema. Pain can also be associated with radiation fibrosis, post-surgical causes and brachial plexus lesions (Vecht 1990) in addition to infection or muscular strain (Badger et al. 1988).

Pain occurring in a limb which has developed lymphoedema is reported to have a number of characteristics which vary according to the underlying cause of the pain (Carroll & Rose 1992).

- The pain is usually exacerbated by activity and relieved by rest.
- The pain is worse at the end of the day and in warm weather.
- The swollen limb feels heavy and aches.
- Comfort and relief are obtained by resting the swollen limb rather than by the use of analgesia.

Twycross (2000) suggests that pain is not just a sensation but a somato-psychic experience influenced by mood and morale. Management of the symptoms of pain should therefore follow a multimodal approach as one or more interventions may reduce or alleviate the individual's pain.

Psychological morbidity

The psychological burden of lymphoedema is clearly documented among breast cancer patients with arm swelling (Tobin et al. 1993, Woods 1993) and many of the issues highlighted can also be considered relevant to those with lymphoedema of the leg, although no formalised research studies on this subject have been completed with this group of patients.

Patients describe a fear that the cancer has recurred when lymphoedema first develops and once lymphoedema has been diagnosed there is a fear that it means that the cancer may recur at some time in the future. In some cases the patient may blame themselves for the development of the swelling, believing it is something they could have avoided.

The swelling serves as a visible reminder of their diagnosis and the treatment completed and, unlike the results of surgery or radiotherapy, it cannot easily be disguised under clothing. Particular difficulties can develop if adaptation is required to aspects of daily life or if function of the limb becomes reduced.

For some, the psychological morbidity associated with the development of lymphoedema causes significant problems and psychological support may be required to enable them to develop coping strategies.

Breast, genital and truncal oedema

Although lymphoedema most commonly affects a limb, it can also involve the adjoining quadrant of the trunk or develop within the breast and genital areas of the body if lymphatic channels in these areas have been influenced by cancer treatment. In patients who have had treatment involving the cervical lymph nodes of the neck, lymphoedema can become problematic in the head and neck region.

Breast oedema

Treatment for breast cancer focuses on conservative management of the axilla and breast. Many patients may then undergo radiation therapy to the breast and supraclavicular areas of the body or reconstructive surgery of the breast. It is not uncommon for patients to experience swelling following these procedures and the affected breast/chest wall can remain swollen for some time. Lymphatic drainage can become impaired and lead to symptoms which include a hardening of the tissues and lymphoedema.

Management of lymphoedema in the breast includes the use of a well-fitting, supportive bra which has deep sides and wide straps to support all breast tissue. The insertion of foam chip pads into the bra can help to soften hardened tissue, but should be used with caution to ensure that the skin does not become sore. Manual lymph drainage can promote lymph drainage from the area and several courses of treatment may be required.

Genital oedema

The development of lymphoedema in genital regions can be very uncomfortable and distressing for patients, affecting personal and sexual relationships. Male patients may experience penile swelling, making micturition difficult, and oedema in the scrotal areas can be painful and embarrassing. There is an increased risk of infection if swelling develops within genital regions and lymphangiomata have a tendency to occur in these areas.

The management of lymphoedema in the genital regions involves a focus on hygiene to minimise the risk of infection and the avoidance of friction during sexual activity. The oedema can be controlled with firm underwear and manual lymphatic drainage to promote lymph drainage from the area.

Truncal oedema

Lymphatic fluid may become trapped in the truncal region following surgical procedures or become transposed from an adjacent swollen limb. Patients may experience sensations of pressure or tightness in the trunk which may be permanent or fluctuate. The oedema may be visible and can be determined with a clinical 'pinch test' in which a fold of tissue is lifted on each side of the chest wall to establish whether there is a difference in texture. Roberts et al. (1995) demonstrated an objective measure of truncal oedema using modified Harpenden skin fold calipers in order to assess changes in swelling.

The management of truncal oedema is aimed at improving patient comfort. Adequate, sustainable compression on the trunk to promote lymph drainage can be provided by specially designed garments and enhanced by the use of manual lymphatic drainage.

Venous complications

The venous and lymphatic systems are closely linked and abnormalities of function in one system will have an impact upon both systems.

Deep vein thrombosis (DVT)

Immobility of a heavy swollen limb can lead to the development of a deep vein thrombosis and the condition can occur despite the wearing of a compression garment. A DVT causes damage to the valves in the veins, resulting in an increase in capillary filtration and a subsequent increase in swelling as the absent or incompetent lymphatics fail to drain.

Altered venous flow

Surgery to remove tumour can alter venous flow and in a study of 81 patients with breast cancer-related arm swelling, only 30% had normal venous outflow demonstrated on colour duplex Doppler imaging (Svensson et al. 1994). Venous outflow complications can cause or exacerbate lymphoedema (Mortimer 2003).

Superior vena caval obstruction

Compression of the upper mediastinal lymph nodes by metastatic disease or secondary venous thrombosis can cause obstruction of the superior vena cava. The symptoms of this complication may develop quickly, are distressing for the patient and, if severe, can be life threatening. The patient may present with swelling in the arm, neck or facial area and describe a feeling of fullness in the head and sensation of choking. Treatment is aimed at reducing the obstruction and providing relief from the associated symptoms.

The following case scenario illustrates the management of lymphorrhoea developing as a complication of lymphoedema.

Case Scenario

Martin is a 40-year-old man who lives with his mother. When he was 28, he developed a lump in his left groin which was found to be due to histiocytosis X, a cancer-like condition in which tumours can develop within the lymph glands. His disease has been controlled with courses of steroids but two years ago he developed another lump in his right groin and despite further treatment with chemotherapy, he developed lymphoedema in both legs and his scrotum.

Martin has been receiving advice and treatment for his lymphoedema which his mother ensures he follows. She asks him to shower each day and puts moisturising cream on his legs and reminds him to put his compression garments on each day before he leaves for work in a local shop. Although his skin tends to be dry and flaky, the swelling has been well controlled and Martin continues to wear his compression garments reluctantly.

Following the death of a close relative, Martin's mother went to Australia for a month. Martin had cared for himself before but during the third week of his mother's absence, he telephoned the clinic to request an appointment because he could not get his stockings on and he had developed a leakage of fluid from his legs which was causing him considerable discomfort and inconvenience. He had been trying to stop the fluid leaking from his legs by using plasters, but these did not stick because his skin was too wet. Martin was also worried because he had not been able to go to work while his legs were leaking so much and he had been sitting at home hoping the leaking would stop. His mother told him on the telephone to make an appointment.

When Martin arrived in the lymphoedema clinic he was distressed by the constant leaking of his legs. The skin of both legs felt cold to the touch and was dry and flaky with lymphorrhoea springing from areas of dryness on the calf area of both legs. His trousers, socks and trainers were wet from the constant leaking.

Reflect on what you know of Martin's history and consider what may have caused the lymphorrhoea to develop in both legs.

- What are Martin's immediate needs?
- How can these be met?

Martin developed lymphorrhoea in both legs because the skin had become excessively dry and hypertrophic. He had not been looking after his legs while his mother had been away and he had wanted to see if he could manage without his compression stockings.

Martin required immediate help to stop the leakage of fluid. This would make him more comfortable, minimise the risk of infection developing in his legs and prevent his skin from breaking down due to the constant moisture. He also required a review of his skin care in order to rehydrate his skin and prevent further trauma. In the longer term, a review of his understanding regarding the management of his lymphoedema and consideration of his compression therapy would be necessary to prevent the situation from happening again.

In order to stop the leakage of fluid, Martin's legs were thoroughly cleansed, dried and moisturised with an emollient, as detailed in Table 12.1. Compression bandages were then applied as detailed in Table 12.2 and Martin was asked to return to the clinic the following day. After 24 hours, the bandages had remained dry but there was some exudate on the dressings next to the skin. The skin was cleansed and moisturised again, prior to reapplication of the bandages. After a further 24 hours there was no further leakage but the bandages were reapplied for a further 24 hours to ensure that the skin condition was improving. After a further 24 hours, Martin was able to be refitted with his compression stockings. At a follow-up appointment with his mother a few weeks later, his skin was considerably better and he continued to wear his compression stockings.

Conclusion

The aim of all health-care professionals should be the early identification and appropriate management of lymphoedema in order to prevent complications from developing. The complications outlined in this chapter can challenge the skills of a specialist and should always be referred for advice and management to the relevant specialist as early as possible. With suitable management and intervention, the patient's quality of life can then be maintained and the lymphoedema controlled.

References

Badger C., Mortimer P., Regnard C. and Twycross R. (1988) Pain in the chronically swollen limb. In: H. Partch (ed.) *Progress in Lymphology*. Elsevier, Netherlands, pp. 243–6.

Carroll D. and Rose K. (1992) Treatment leads to significant improvement: effect of conservative treatment on pain in lymphoedema. *Professional Nurse*, 8(1): 32–6.

Foldi E. and Foldi M. (2003) Lymphostatic diseases. In: M. Foldi, E. Foldi and S. Kubik (eds) *Textbook of Lymphology for Physicians and Lymphoedema Therapists*. Urban and Fischer, Germany, pp. 232–319.

International Society of Lymphology (2000) The diagnosis and treatment of peripheral lymphoedema. Consensus document of the International Society of Lymphology. *Lymphology*, 36(2): 84–91.

Ling J., Duncan A., Laverty D. and Hardy J. (1997) Lymphorrhoea in palliative care. *European Journal of Palliative Care*, **4**(2): 50–2.

Linnett N. (2000) Skin management in lymphoedema. In: R. Twycross, K. Jenns and J. Todd (eds) *Lymphoedema*. Radcliffe Medical Press, Oxford, pp. 118–29.

Maclaren J. (2001) Skin changes in lymphoedema: pathophysiology and management options. *International Journal of Palliative Nursing*, **7**(8): 381–8.

Melzack R. (1975) The McGill Pain Questionnaire. *Pain*, **1**(3): 277–99.

Mortimer P. (2003) Lymphoedema of the upper limb. In: N. Browse, K. Burnand and P. Mortimer (eds) *Diseases of the Lymphatics*. Arnold/Oxford University Press, London, pp. 231–42.

Mulvenna P., Gillham L. and Regnard C. (1995) Lymphangiosarcomata–experience in a lymphoedema clinic. *Palliative Medicine*, **9**(1): 55–9.

Roberts C., Levick J., Stanton A. and Mortimer P. (1995) Assessment of truncal oedema following breast cancer treatment using modified Harpenden skinfold callipers. *Lymphology*, **28**(2): 78–88.

Sitzia J. and Sobrido L. (1997) Measurement of health-related quality of life of patients receiving conservative treatment for limb lymphoedema using the Nottingham Health Profile. *Quality of Life Research*, **6**(5): 373–84.

Svensson W., Mortimer P., Tohno E. and Cosgrove D. (1994) Colour Doppler demonstrates venous flow abnormalities in breast cancer patients with chronic arm swelling. *European Journal of Cancer*, **30**(5): 657–60.

Tobin M., Lacey H., Meyer L. and Mortimer P. (1993) The psychological morbidity of breast cancer related arm swelling. *Cancer*, **72**(11): 3248–52.

Twycross R. (2000) Pain in lymphoedema. In: R. Twycross, K. Jenns and J. Todd (eds) *Lymphoedema*. Radcliffe Medical Press, Oxford, pp. 68–88.

Vecht C. (1990) Arm pain in the patient with breast cancer. *Journal of Pain and Symptom Management*, **5**(2): 109–17.

Williams A. (2004) Understanding and managing lymphoedema in people with advanced cancer. *Journal of Clinical Nursing*, **18**(11): 32–7.

Woods M. (1993) Patients' perceptions of breast cancer related lymphoedema. *European Journal of Cancer Care*, **2**: 125–8.

Woods M. (2004) External compression and support in the management of lymphoedema. In: L. Dougherty and S. Lister (eds) *The Royal Marsden Hospital Manual of Clinical Nursing Procedures*, 6th edn. Blackwell, Oxford, pp. 348–61.

Glossary of Terms

Acute lymphoedema Swelling that develops immediately or within the first 6–8 weeks post treatment which is usually painless, mild and transient.

Body image A person's impression of how their body looks.

Brachial plexopathy Progressive loss of sensation and motor function in the arm associated with radiation treatment involving the brachial nerve.

British Lymphology Society A registered charity established to provide support and education to all health-care professionals, as well as others, who are directly involved in the management of lymphoedema.

Chronic lymphoedema Lymphoedema that is present over a long period of time and causes a long-term change in the body.

Compression bandages Low-stretch bandages used as the outer layer of a multilayer system of bandages and padding to provide a semi-rigid encasement to the swollen limb with the aim of reducing limb volume or reshaping a swollen limb.

Compression garments Sleeves, stockings or other body garments produced to a standard or custom-made shape for a patient to wear on a regular basis with the aim of controlling their lymphoedema.

Cording Tender cord-like structures of varying thickness which develop postoperatively and occur most frequently along the arm following breast cancer surgery.

Emollients Bland, unperfumed skin moisturisers or soap substitutes applied daily to promote integrity of the superficial layer of the skin and enhance hydration.

Fibrosis A thickening of connective tissue which indicates an end-stage in normal pathological processes as a result of lymph stasis in the tissues.

Filariasis Lymphoedema, endemic to the tropics, caused by a parasitic tissue-dwelling worm which enters the body via the vector of a mosquito.

Folliculitis Tiny spots appearing on the skin from inflammation of the hair follicle caused by the use of greasy moisturisers which have become trapped within the hair follicle.

Hyperkeratosis A build-up of horny skin which leads to a warty, thickened appearance with skin creases.

Incidence The number of new cases of a disease developing in a defined population over a specified period of time.

Intensive phase of treatment A short, planned period of therapist-led daily lymphoedema treatment with clear aims and objectives for the outcome.

Ipsilateral Lymphoedema involving one limb, as compared to bilateral which means both limbs.

Isometric exercises The muscle length remains unchanged during muscular contraction.

Isotonic exercises The muscle is lengthened or shortened during muscular contraction.

Latency stage of lymphoedema A variable time period following the resolution of acute swelling during which the person remains at risk of the further development of lymphoedema.

Limb volume measurements Multiple circumferential measurements taken of both limbs at 4 cm intervals and applied to the formula for the volume of a cylinder to determine the excess volume of the swollen limb.

Lymphangioma Extremely dilated lymphatic vessels in the superficial dermis which bulge on the skin, causing the appearance of a blister.

Lymphatic system A one-way drainage system which defends the body against infection and absorbs cell debris.

Lymphoedema Support Network A national patient organisation which is a registered charity established to provide information, support and advice for those affected by lymphoedema.

Lymphorrhoea The development of lymph fluid leaking through the skin in a limb or area where swelling is present.

Maintenance phase of treatment A self-care phase of treatment in which the person with lymphoedema adopts responsibility for the long-term control of their swelling by managing it on a daily basis.

Manual lymphatic drainage (MLD) A form of skin massage in which specialised hand movements are used by a trained therapist in a systematic, repetitive manner to manually stimulate movement of lymph fluid within the lymphatic channels.

Objective assessment An assessment based on measurable facts which are free from personal opinion or feelings.

Oedema Tissue swelling which develops when the volume of fluid entering the interstitial compartment of the tissues is greater than the rate at which it is drained.

Olecranon A bony prominence which can be located at the elbow and is the end of the ulna bone in the forearm.

Papillomatosis Papules or nodules, caused by dilated skin lymphatics surrounded by rigid fibrous tissue which protrude from the surface of the skin to give a cobblestone appearance.

Patella A thick triangular bone, known as the kneecap, which covers and protects the knee joint.

Prevalence The number of cases of a disease existing in a given population at one point in time.

Primary lymphoedema Lymphoedema arising from a congenital abnormality, occurring within the lymphatic system.

Secondary lymphoedema Lymphoedema developing as a result of an external influence affecting the function of the lymphatic system.

Seroma An accumulation of serous fluid at the wound site after surgery which sometimes requires aspiration with a needle.

Simple lymphatic drainage (SLD) Simple self-massage movements based on the principles of manual lymph drainage which are carried out by the patient or carer on areas of normal lymph drainage.

Simple surface measurements Measurements of a limb taken with a tape measure at three or four points along the length of the limb to indicate its size and enable broad changes to be identified over time.

Stemmer's sign A positive indication that lymphoedema is present based on an inability to pick up a fold of skin at the base of the toes or fingers.

Subjective assessment An assessment based on personal opinion or observation rather than scientific measurement.

Thrombosis The coagulation of blood in a blood vessel.

Trigger factors Actions or behaviours which may initiate the development of lymphoedema in a limb at risk of its development following treatment involving the lymph nodes.

Venepuncture The insertion of a needle into a vein for therapeutic purposes.

Useful Addresses and Websites

Patient information and advice

Breast Cancer Care
Kiln House, 210 New Kings Road, London SW6 4NZ
Tel: 020 7384 2984
www.breastcancercare.org.uk
Booklet entitled 'Living with Lymphoedema after Breast Cancer Treatment' available on request or to download via the website.

Cancerbacup
3 Bath Place, Rivington Street, London WC2A 3JR
Tel: 0808 800 1234
www.cancerbacup.org.uk
Booklet entitled 'Understanding Lymphoedema' available upon request or to download via the website.

CancerHelp UK
Tel: 0800 226 237
www.cancerhelp.org.uk
Free website information about cancer which includes information about lymphoedema.

Lymphoedema Association of Australia
www.lymphoedema.org.au
Patient support group in Australia.

Lymphedema People
www.lymphedemapeople.com
Information on the causes and treatment of lymphoedema plus articles and
a discussion forum.

Lymphoedema Support Network
St Lukes Crypt, Sydney Street, London SW3 6NH
Tel: 020 7351 4480
www.lymphoedema.org/lsn
A variety of leaflets and videos for patients prepared by health-care professionals on different aspects of lymphoedema, telephone helpline and
support groups.

National Lymphedema Network
www.lymphnet.org
Patient support group in America.

NHS Direct Online Health Encyclopaedia
www.nhsdirect.org
Advice on the prevention of lymphoedema available via the website.

Royal Marsden NHS Foundation Trust
Fulham Road, London SW3 6JJ
Tel: 020 7352 8171
www.royalmarsden.org
Comprehensive patient information leaflets and booklets on lymphoedema
for cancer patients which can be purchased or accessed through the Patient
Information section of the website.

Skin Care Campaign
www.skincarecampaign.org
Information leaflet on lymphoedema available on the website in the
'Directory of Skin Diseases'.

Health-care professional information and advice

Activa Health Care
1 Lancaster Park, Newborough Road, Needwood, Burton-upon-Trent,
Staffordshire DE13 9PD
Tel: 08450 606707
www.activahealthcare.co.uk
A company that offers complete compression therapy solutions.

British Lymphology Society
PO Box 196, Shoreham, Sevenoaks TN13 9BF
www.lymphoedema.org/bls
The website provides information and advice on aspects of lymphoedema service provision and management. There is an annual conference and regional representative network to co-ordinate local activities for lymphoedema therapists.

BSN Medical Ltd
PO Box 258, Willerby, Hull HU10 6WT
Tel: 01482 670100
www.bsnmedical.com
BSN Medical offers a complete range of bandage products, paddings and compression garments for professional bandaging of oedematous limbs.

Credenhill Ltd
10 Cossall Industrial Estate, Ilkeston, Derbyshire DE7 5UG
Tel: 0115 932 0144
www.credenhill.co.uk
Credenhill is a specialist distributor of compression hosiery and complementary equipment, supplying hospitals and pharmacies across the UK with products to suit the needs of every patient.

Haddenham Healthcare Ltd
Crendon House, Crendon Industrial Park, Long Crendon, Buckinghamshire HP18 9BB
Tel: 01844 208842
www.hadhealth.com
A company offering a range of patient-friendly products for lymphoedema, breast care and vascular patients.

Juzo UK Ltd
Unit 1, Edison Place, Dryburgh Industrial Estate, Dundee DD2 3QU
Tel: 01382 826620
www.juzo.com
An international company providing medical compression therapy garments.

Medi UK Ltd
Plough Lane, Hereford HR4 0EL
Tel: 01432 373500
www.mediuk.co.uk
A company providing a range of vascular, lymphoedema and orthopaedic products to the medical profession.

Sigvaris Britain Ltd
The Foundry, London Road, Kingsworthy, Winchester SO23 7QD
Tel: 01264 326666
www.sigvaris.com
The Sigvaris product range comprises medical compression stockings for the treatment and support stockings for the prevention of lymphatic and venous disorders as well as innovative products for improving quality of life.

Further Reading

Journal of Lymphoedema
Biannual journal for improving practice, raising awareness and setting standards for care.
Published by Wounds UK, Aberdeen AB10 1BA
Tel: 01224 637 371

Lymphoedema Bandaging in Practice (2005)
European Wound Management Association (EWMA) Focus Document
Published by Medical Education Partnership (MEP) Ltd, 53 Hargrave Road, London N19 5SH
Tel: 020 7561 5400

Template for Practice: Compression Hosiery in Lymphoedema (2006)
Published by Medical Education Partnership (MEP) Ltd, 53 Hargrave Road, London N19 5SH
Tel: 020 7561 5400

International Consensus: Best Practice for the Management of Lymphoedema (2006)
Published by Medical Education Partnership (MEP) Ltd, 53 Hargrave Road, London N19 5SH
Tel: 020 7561 5400

Index